SCOFF-NOSH

PALEO

151 + Delicious PALEO RECIPES FOR

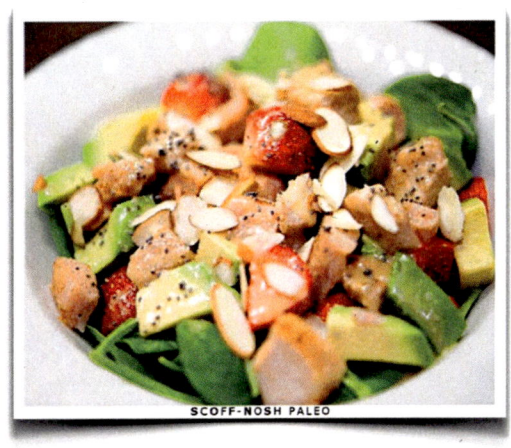

SCOFF-NOSH PALEO

MODERN DAY "HUNTER GATHERERS"

Delicious

RECIPES FREE FROM

WHEAT - GLUTEN – SUGAR– GRAINS - LEGUMES & DAIRY

OLIVER MICHAELS

PALAEO-

ˈPALɪəʊˈ, ˈPEɪLɪəʊˈ/
COMBINING FORM
PREFIX: PALEO-

Older or ancient, especially relating to the
geological past "Palaeolithic".

The Paleolithic diet commonly referred to as the caveman diet, Stone Age diet
and the hunter-gatherer diet.

This diet is a modern nutritional plan based on the scientific research and
presumed ancient diet. The diet consisted of wild plants, fruits, nuts and lean
natural grass fed animal meats.

This was a period of about 2.6 million years that ended around 10,000 years ago
with the development of the agricultural revolution and grain-based diets.

In 1985 S. Boyd Eaton and Melvin Konner, both of Emory University, published a
paper on Paleolithic nutrition in the New England Journal of Medicine, this
attracted the wider mainstream medical attention.

This diet has gathered so much momentum and popularity over the past few years
since it was introduced.

In common usage, the term "paleolithic diet" can also refer to actual ancestral
human diets, insofar as these diets are translated and can be reconstructed.

SCOFF-NOSH

PALEO

151 + DELICIOUS PALEO RECIPES FOR MODERN DAY "HUNTER GATHERERS".

Printed in the United States of America

ISBN -13: 978-1497396029

ISBN -10: 1497396026

printedition viii.ix 2014 ©.

FOR MORE INFORMATION GO TO: - Oliver Michaels Author Central on Amazon.

Other Books by the
AUTHOR

The Green Juice Detox Diet. AMAZING HEALTHY GREEN JUICE RECIPES AND MORE..

The Green Juice Recipe Book. amazon *#1 Best Seller*

JUST AMAZING HEALTHY GREEN JUICE RECIPES…

The Green Juice Recipe Book for Kids &

Family Health.

AMAZING DELICIOUS JUICE RECIPES & HEALTHY LIVING FOR KIDS AND THE WHOLE FAMILY.

41 Miracle Juice recipes For Men's Health

THE REVOLUTIONARY JUICING PLAN FOR GETTING LEAN, BUILDING MUSCLE AND HEALTHY VIBRANT SKIN…

41 Miracle Beauty Juice Recipes. DISCOVER THE TOP ANTI-AGING SUPERFOODS FOR RADIANT SKIN, HEALTH AND FAST WEIGHT LOSS. …

COMING SOON
Email olivermichaels.author@hotmail.com "FREE" to get NEW Healthy eBOOK Releases FREE **Coming SOON!**

TABLE OF CONTENTS

PREFACE.

Best Selling Author Oliver Michaels takes us on his journey for the ultimate balance of modern living while enjoying a healthy diet with his simple, healthy and nutritious Paleo Diet Cookbook **SCOFF NOSH PALEO**.

This diet is based on the ideas that all healthy and nutritious foods are not processed in a packet, or consumed in a wonder pill. Instead your healthy food comes directly from the land. Inside this stylish cookbook Oliver will help you to embrace healthy paleo food, while maintaining your busy and modern lifestyle.

"I have studied the paleo diet, benefits and science for the past 5 years, eating paleo food is my chosen diet with the addition of my daily juice supplements. The healthy principle of Paleo food forms the main part of my overall health regime. I find paleo serves every health benefit it professes to. I want to share with you my experiences, the benefits, and everything Paleo, showing you how to gain the best results from your new paleo lifestyle.

My goal is to provide you with all the information you need to discover and fully enjoy this natural way of food. I have included over 151+ healthy recipes, Including, benefits of using herbs, Paleo Snacks on the go!, (recipes that allow you to still enjoy paleo food, (even with your modern busy lifestyle).

So come back to our basics, regain your health and eat the natural nutritional foods our genes require for our health, this is the diet we have eaten for the past 2.6 million years, and has been missing for over 10,000 years.

I sincerely hope you enjoy this Cook Book, and go on to love your Healthy Paleo life style and delicious Paleo food".

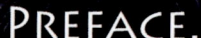

SCOFF NOSH PALEO

How to use this Paleo Cookbook.

I hope you find this book as easy to follow as I have intended, I've divided it into 3 easy to follow sections, over 18 chapters crammed with paleo info and delicious recipes.

CHAPTERS 1 - 5: - See your diet throughout evolution, understanding what we are designed to eat. Journey through our paleo, agricultural and modern day GMO diet....

CHAPTERS 6 - 7: - Preparing for paleo the do's and don'ts. Stocking your pantry. Realizing the benefits of cutting out Processed Foods, see how easy, delicious and enjoyable paleo food really is...

CHAPTERS 8 - 18: - Finally prepare, discover and create the delicious mouth-watering paleo recipes and snacks
All 151+ of them.

Most of the recipes rely on your cooking with vegetables, meats, spices, and fats to allow your taste buds to party within the nature of paleo. Eating paleo gets you away from the nonsense of traditional calorie and points counting diets.

Fat is an essential nutrient for energy and health, but it is so important to flavour your food too, remember there's no calorie counting or dieting when we eat food as nature intended.

I have tried to keep these recipes as simple as possible while not compromising on taste. While keeping the choice of recipes varied, some are quick and simple some more slightly involved family meals. Your slow cooker will earn its keep too!

You will see I have included prep times, and cooking times with yield.

Cooking these tasty healthy recipes is a super way to socialize and enjoy food with your friends and family.

I also want to minimize your time cooking and maximize your time enjoying amazing healthy food.

Everyone should at least try paleo food, even if you try just one recipe. By engaging just one element of the paleo lifestyle towards your regular food diet, is to make a huge step in the right direction for good health.

Consuming healthy, non-processed foods as nature intended is, exactly what it is, Paleo!

Oliver Michaels

INTRODUCTION

I consume all non-processed food, I am on a gluten – sugar – grain – legume, alcohol and dairy FREE DIET. Ok then YES, just an occasional drop of alcohol

My diet has been successful and very healthy through using the 80 - 20 rule (more about this later *).

After my body's non-acceptance of dairy and processed food (along with a whopping 65% of the world's population), I endured years of suffering with digestion issues, stomach bloating and ill health. I was later diagnosed with lactose intolerance.

I have written this book to share with you the incredible health benefits, delicious healthy recipes, and the foundation of the diet of the Paleolithic man and woman.

Over the past 3 years I wanted to know if the paleo diet was in fact healthy. Throughout this cookbook you will discover some amazing nutritional evidence, some common sense, some healthy motivators and some REAL *"ah-ha"* moments. All with up to date research that supports the delicious recipes of this amazing evolutionary food.

What I share with you leaves me with NO DOUBT as to what diet we should ALL be eating today.

*The Paleo diet is the diet that I live by using the 80 - 20 rule, 80% of the time I EAT a 100% Paleo diet, with a 20% margin for straying outside. This does happen, less often than it did initially, but it takes ALL pressure away from diet failure.

Today I have NO health concerns and lead a healthy active life. I no longer ignore the effects of processed food on my health and wellness. The undeniable evidence is that through eating processed foods and factory-produced meat, we are ingesting chemicals that are making us ALL sick!

The paleo diet is one of the fastest growing diets today, why? because Paleo is backed with nutritional scientific evidence. Our evolution has shown we have only become chronically sick over the past 50 - 100 years of eating highly processed food and unethically raised livestock meat.

Lets be honest with ourselves, we have all tried eating healthier foods, we then end up back in our same eating habits several weeks, or even days later.

The fast pace of modern living, convenience foods, restaurants and 24hr fast food, all takes a daily bite ☺ out of our diet discipline. This eventually takes us down that unhealthy eating route back into our old habits.

What seems like a good idea in principle soon fades into what I call, our 'Every Day Reality'.

The paleo diet isn't about starving yourself, in fact it's quite the opposite. This diet involves a complete over indulgence of nutrition including phytonutrients, healthy fats, protein and essential amino acids that your body requires. Eat delicious healthy foods until you are satisfied and see the unwanted weight fall off and enjoy a new feeling of energy, health and vitality.

It is hard to resist the addictive properties that processed and heavily marketed healthy food has been engineered to do. I will be honest, it is something I did battle with early on, but there is a difference, I am prepared and willing to win this battle and not end up another unhealthy statistic.

I've tackled, head on the outrageous methods of modern processed foods, and researched the incredible diet of our ancestors and how the ignorance and greed of man has been so badly translated into today. Since Paleo, our food has been largely unchanged, over the past 10,000 years, since the agricultural revolution. However, over the past 50 years food has been heavily produced by genetically modified processes, containing toxic and highly addictive chemicals, this being the main cause of increased diet related diseases today.

Over 70% of the average western diet is processed food, with over 80% of the processed food in the US being banned in other nations. [1] The increase in childhood and adult obesity, diabetes and heart disease is at an all time high at 45%. [3]

By 2040 it is estimated over 70% of Americans will outlive their children, and / or die from obesity themselves. [4] I am looking at our diet from the hard facts and the greed of only a few companies who are now controlling how our food is produced, or should I say genetically modified. Even if you don't eat in fast food restaurants you are not off the hook, the food you are buying is produced to the fast food production standard. One of the largest fast food chains dictate how our food is produced, being the largest purchaser of Beef, Pork, Chicken, Potatoes, Lettuce and Tomatoes In the world!

Yes, even our vegetables and fruit like, tomatoes are picked prematurely developed, lacking major nutritional content from sunlight and natural growth. Instead, they are picked for their maximum shelf life and before transportation, they are sprayed with ethane gas to ripen them. Beef fillers are sprayed with ammonia to kill e-coli and livestock cattle are fed genetically modified corn, hormones and steroids for fast growth, not to mention inhumane slaughter.

Chickens who never see daylight are fed steroids, hormones and antibiotics to kill the spread of infections and bacteria. Their growth is accelerated from the normal healthy 70 days to adulthood, to just 40 days before they are sent to the factory and killed.

We are now living in a world of GMO food manufacturing. We are no longer naturally growing crops or raising livestock. Corporations like Monsanto, Tyson, and Smithfield have the monopoly on how all food is processed. They continue to badly affect our health, quality of life, our life span and now that of our children.

Chapters One - Five

Blueberries are a popular paleo food choice and can be added to so many recipes... These tiny berries are a nutrtional POWER HOUSE full of vitamin C, as well as manganese. They are also a great source of fiber, which is an important copmponent of keeping your heart healthy and your cholesterol low. Blueberries are also one of the Best sources of antioxidants.

CHAPTER 1

WHAT IS THE PALEO DIET?

If man and woman, really are the most intelligent species on earth, then why do we eat food genetically modified with zero nutritional value and laced with poisonous chemicals and pesticides?

The Paleolithic diet, also called the "Caveman" or "Stone Age" diet, is based around the idea that we should eat like our ancestors did over 2.6 million years ago. This is a massive total of 99.6 % of our evolutionary history, and why our genome (The genome is the entirety of an organism's hereditary information), has been perfectly adapted to eat foods similar to what we found during that period of time. We therefore will live a healthier life, live longer, maintain healthy weight and curb disease.

So this means foods that can be hunted or gathered like fish, meat, shellfish, poultry, eggs, veggies, roots, fruits and berries should be consumed.

However, the paleo diet consists of no grains, no dairy, no legumes (beans or peas), no refined or artificial sugar or salt, (unless unrefined iodized sea salt which has trace minerals) and no alcohol.

OUR EVOLUTIONARY TIME ON EARTH IN A 24 HOUR CLOCK TIME PERIOD: -

23:54:06 hrs.

PALEOLITHIC MANS genome, (Genes and DNA) responsible for our human survival. **This has evolved over the past 23 hours 54 minutes and 6 seconds.**

00:05:51 hrs.

The AGRICULTURAL REVOLUTION This see's the introduction of farming animals, grain and wheat. **This has evolved over the past 5 minutes and 51 seconds.**

00:00:03 hrs.

GMO & PROCESSED FOOD has been produced. This food is now predominantly consumed worldwide. **This has evolved over the past 3 seconds.**

SO WHY IS PALEO FOOD MORE HEALTHY?

Over the past 2.6 million years we all know our bodies have been genetically predisposed to eat this way. Millions of years of our human evolution has shaped us the way we are today.

Our shift from paleo food is due to the development of the agricultural revolution, approximately (10,000 years ago). This led to a dramatic change in human nutrition. The introduction of cereal grains, legumes, dairy, vegetable oils, salt, alcohol, and refined sugars. This now comprises about 72% of the food consumption in the western diet. These recent additions to the human diet maintain nutritional characteristics that promote virtually all known diseases of our civilization.

Additionally, over the past 50 years we saw the birth of gmo and mass processed food production. Food that is not grown through traditional methods, the increase in grain and modified soy in our diets, this has all wreaked havoc on our health.

This includes the huge onset of chronic diseases like obesity, heart disease, cancers and diabetes.

Eating the healthy Paleo diet encourages us to consume more fruit, vegetables, healthy fats and proteins and cut out added sugars and salts.

The combination of plant food nutrients, phytonutrients, omega 3 and a diet rich in fats and protein can help control our blood sugars, provide energy and regulate our bodies.

Since starting the paleo diet I have had moments of straying from my paleo food. This is down to foods like the smell of regular cookies with their enticing aroma and consumer-enticing packaging. I will be honest it was sometimes more than I could handle. I have sometimes asked myself the question

"Wait, why am I not eating grains again?"

This part is dedicated to you, if you have the same temptations in your live and in your food cupboards, as I did. Yes, I too needed the reminder of why I ate a paleo diet.

The key to paleo is the snack food, in fact, with any diet, you need to have the right snack at hand that are healthy, tasty and nutritious. I discovered and created some amazing **paleo snack, 'on the go recipes'.** See **Chapter 8** for these delicious healthy recipes.

It's can be confusing that grains and legumes (all beans – black, pinto, soy, peanuts, etc.) Would be so pleasing to us, since there makeup is dependent on plant reproductive survival, making them basically poisonous to humans. They contribute heavily to the current, overwhelming predominance of heart disease, digestive disorders and obesity rates in the western world.

There are many reasons for this, grains and legumes contain an unsavoury collection of "anti-nutrients". Some of them strip away your body's mineral reserves, cause intestinal damage and also problems to your immunity levels. Lets briefly look at the little anti-nutrient proteins called lectins.

WHAT ARE LECTINS?

Lectins are proteins found in all animals (including us) and in plants too, especially in grains, legumes (especially soy), but also nuts and seeds. They have many protective functions in the human body, from recognizing pathogens to controlling protein levels in our blood. Their function in plants is also protective, to the plant that is!

Lectins are found in the seeds of plants and they have a function towards the survival of the seed. The way they protect the seed is that they can cause considerable intestinal distress (bloating, diarrhoea, nausea, vomiting, even death) to those who eat the seeds. This then deters the predator from coming back for more, its part of the plant evolution, reproduction and survival.

Wheat contains a lectin called wheat germ agglutinin (WGA). These lectins are a sticky consistency and they go into your small intestine and gloms onto the brush border, (the membrane of the small intestine). This then tricks your body into taking it across the membrane of your intestine intact. Here it is seen as a foreign invader by your immune system. Antibodies are created in response to these lectins.

Unfortunately, they often look a lot like other cells of your body, cells in your brain, pancreas, etc. So the same antibodies that were created to attack the lectins will actually go launch attacks on your own body. This is where autoimmune issues arise, like diabetes type 1, celiac disease, lupus and multiple sclerosis.

LEAKY GUT .

Further to the above, on their way into your body, lectins damage the walls of your intestines. This causes what we know as "leaky gut", so that other larger particles can cross the intestinal barrier, enter your blood stream and develop other immune problems including food sensitivities. Something goes in (like the WGA) and makes some holes in your gut that lets big particles of food into your blood stream. Then your immune system gets VERY overwhelmed and confused and starts attacking things at random.

Symptoms can range from migraine, rashes, inflammation and headaches to eczema, weight gain and depression.

Can you cook Lectins out of the foods?

Cooking, sprouting or soaking your grains, legumes, nuts and seeds can help to decrease the number of lectins they contain, but NONE of those processes totally eliminates the lectins. These are ALL highly heat resistant. They're also resistant to enzymatic activity. Enzymatic activity refers to the action of a particular enzyme on its target. For example, the enzyme called protease in the stomach has an enzymatic action of breaking down proteins. This is why they are so difficult for us, and even our pets to digest.

So should I eat nuts and seeds?

Our ancestors did not have access to a whole bunch of nuts and seeds every day. The reason that nuts and seeds are allowed on this diet but not grains and legumes, is that grains and legumes contain a whole host of other "anti-nutrients" beyond just lectins. *(See My findings page 49 Paleo Diet Nuts)*

Most vegans and vegetarians rely upon legumes, beans, soy, lentils and peas, etc. They also rely on whole grains in an attempt to meet the majority of their daily caloric intake. Legumes and whole grains contain some of the highest concentrations of anti-nutrients than any other foods. These compounds are 'Protease inhibitors' substances that inhibit the actions of trypsin, pepsin and other proteases in the gut. This prevents the digestion and more critically the subsequent absorption of protein.

An example is Bowman-Birk trypsin inhibitor, this is found in soybeans. Their consumption frequently increases intestinal permeability, this is also a cause of "leaky gut," a necessary first step in almost all autoimmune diseases. Furthermore, a leaky gut likely underlies chronic, low-grade inflammation, which cause not only autoimmune diseases, but also heart disease and cancers.

Further to this consuming a vegan and vegetarian diet only, almost invariably result in numerous vitamin, mineral and nutrient deficiencies such as B12, B6, D, zinc, iron, iodine, taurine and omega-3 fatty acids.

Believe it or not these are a delicious and healthy alternative to French Fries.

For this Simple recipe and more go to page 125 & 126

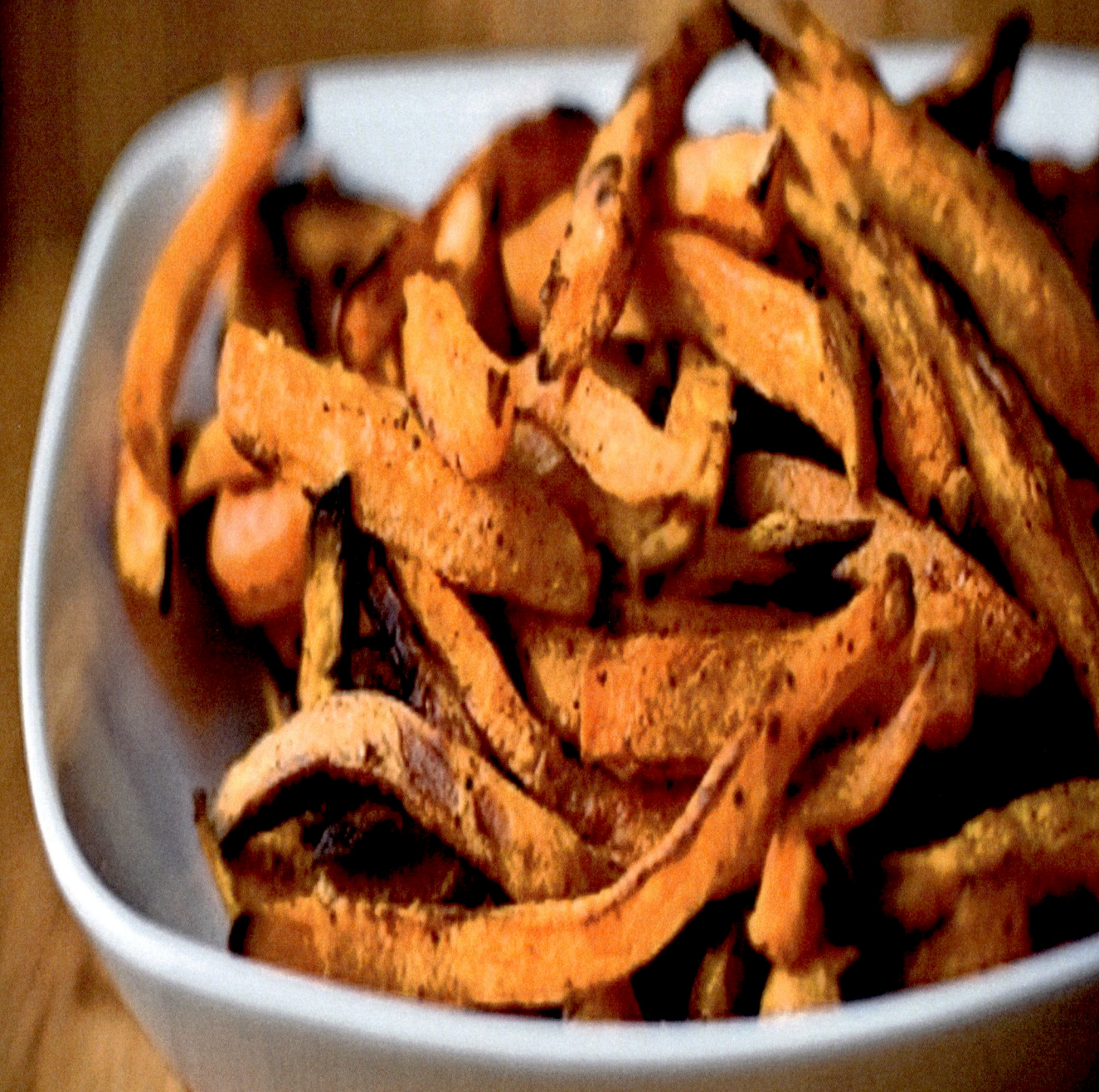

SCOFF-NOS**H** PALEO

CHAPTER 2

IS MAN THE SICKEST ANIMAL ON THE PLANET?

Paleolithic man and woman survive and then progressively adapts to severe environmental changes. We continue to develop over millions of years of evolution to become the most advanced and dominant species on the planet. We are indeed top of the food chain.

Since the evolution of farming and agriculture we have developed techniques and practices to become self-sufficient, raise crops, introducing what was thought to be healthy wheat grain and animal food for a sustainable diet.

Over the past 10,000 years our food has not changed, over this past 50 years our farmed and processed foods have continued to cause havoc to our health as a whole. What we know as metabolic Syndrome, a medical term for a combination of diabetes, high blood pressure and obesity. This is putting us at greater risk of heart disease, stroke and other conditions affecting blood vessels.

"We have become so detached from the very foods that allowed us to be come a highly evolved species".

DAIRY.

Why are we the only mammal on the planet that will drink the milk from another species? 65% of us *(the most intelligent species on the planet)* can't digest the lactose in the milk. This process of lactose intolerance causes severe digestion pain, swelling bloating and discomfort!

Milk is a potent stimulator designed to cause growth in calfs! Milk is reported by scientific research in Scandinavia to be insulin resistant and can help cause and develop obesity. Milk protein, the lactose contains galactose that we DO NOT EAT! Through research milk is linked to prostate cancer in men and ovarian cancer in women. This area is still being researched.

A fellow British health food advocate and world re-known chef gives an amazing impactive speech available on **TED,** where he talks about our diet and the amount of added refined sugar in milk. After the pasturisation process, which kills all nutrients that were present, sugar is then added (5 teaspoons per 250 ml glass). Milk is then packaged as HEALTHY and consumed by millions of us every day and alarmingly largely by our children.

POULTRY.

It is sad to see mans cruelty to other animals to support our food requirements. Food that is raised so unethically that its is truly bad for our health, yet we all have consumed this very food.

Its hard to believe but chickens have quite an impressive lifespan. The maximum age of a chicken is about 25 years. This is rare for them to live that long as they are so vulnerable to predators and disease.

Due to this the average age of a backyard chicken is about 4 years, although with special protection and care it would not be unreasonable to expect 7 or 8 years.

Virtually all chickens raised for their flesh spend their lives crammed into huge windowless sheds that typically hold as many as tens of thousands of birds each.

Chickens normally function well in groups of up to about 90, a number low enough to allow each bird to find there own spot in the pecking order. In crowded groups of tens of thousands no such social order is possible, and in their frustration, they relentlessly peck at each other causing injury and death.

The intense confinement and extreme crowding on large-scale factory farms also results in unimaginable filth and disease. The dust, feathers and ammonia choke the air in the chicken houses. They are then forced to breathe ammonia and particulate matter from faeces and feathers all day long.

Many of them suffer from chronic respiratory diseases, weakened immune systems, bronchitis and ammonia burn.

In 2006 and again in 2010 a study by Consumer Reports [9] found that a huge 85% of food market chickens tested, were infected with either campylobacter or salmonella or both bacteria.

Chickens are fed large quantities of powerful antibiotics to keep them alive in conditions that would otherwise kill them.

Did You Know? Chickens are given nearly four times the amount of antibiotics as human beings or cattle in the United States.

Chickens are also genetically manipulated and regularly dosed with drugs to make them grow faster and larger. The average breast of an 8-week-old chicken is seven times heavier today, than it was 25 years ago. Because of the unnatural accelerated weight gain, these young birds frequently die of heart attacks and lung collapses. This is something that would almost never happen in nature.

Chickens now grow so rapidly that the heart and lungs are not even developed well enough to support the remainder of their body. This results in congestive heart failure and tremendous death losses.

In addition, chickens on today's factory farms almost always become crippled because their legs cannot support the weight of their bodies. In fact, by the age of 6 weeks, 90 percent of chickens are so obese that they can no longer walk. They are sat in their faeces for the remainder of their life before they are slaughtered. Many crippled chickens on factory farms die when they can no longer reach their water.

"We then eat this very food that has been so unethically raised".

Yes, we are indeed top of the food chain. However, this does not mean we should mistreat animals that are providing us food. Cause unnecessary suffering and produce foods that cause us ill health…

MEAT

Intense animal farming practices involve very large numbers of animals raised on limited land that require large amounts of food, water and medical inputs, antibiotic, hormones and steroids to accelerate their growth. These measures are required to keep the animals alive in cramped conditions.

Very large or confined indoor intensive livestock operations (particularly descriptive of common US farming practices) are often referred to as factory farming. Unfortunately and more often then not this can mean a low level of animal welfare standards. The associated pollution to the animal (soon to be our food) includes diseases and major health issues.

The natural food of grass fed cattle and livestock is no longer part of the mass-produced meat production. Grass is not part of their diet, instead they are fed genetically modified soy and corn feeds.

For size and growth they are fed with hormones and steroids to produce a bigger animal for slaughter.

VEGETABLES AND FRUIT

Recent government pesticide tests reveal the widespread presence of pesticide residues on conventionally grown, non-organic fruits and vegetables and even our tap water.

The results analysed by the Environmental Working Group (EWG) show that 68 % of food samples had detectable pesticide residues after they had been washed or peeled.

As a result of the data generated by scientists at U.S. Department of Agriculture and Food and Drug Administration, the working group created the list of foods most commonly contaminated with pesticides.

- 98 % of conventional apples has detectable levels of pesticides.
- Domestic blueberries tested positive for 42 different pesticide residues.
- 78 different pesticides were found on lettuce samples.
- Every single nectarine USDA tested had pesticide residues.
- As a category, grapes generally have more types of pesticides than any other fruit tested. There were 64 different chemicals found in this category.
- 13 different pesticides were measured on a single sample each of celery and strawberries.
- Green beans and leafy greens (kale and collard greens) were commonly contaminated with highly toxic organophosphate insecticides.

These insecticides are known to affect our nervous system.
The produce LEAST likely to test positive for pesticides is asparagus, avocado, cabbage, grapefruit, watermelon, eggplants, pineapples, mushrooms, onions, frozen peas and sweet potatoes.

I don't expect us to be buying all our meat raised organically, grass-fed, pastured, wild, or free-range. I do understand as families we all have a food budget. However buying more ethically raised livestock is better for the animal and also our health. I am saying buy the highest quality of protein you can afford.

We are indeed top of the food chain, and with that comes a responsibility. A responsibility to not only maintain our health and continue our development, but a responsibility to respect and raise all our food ethically.

Oliver Michaels

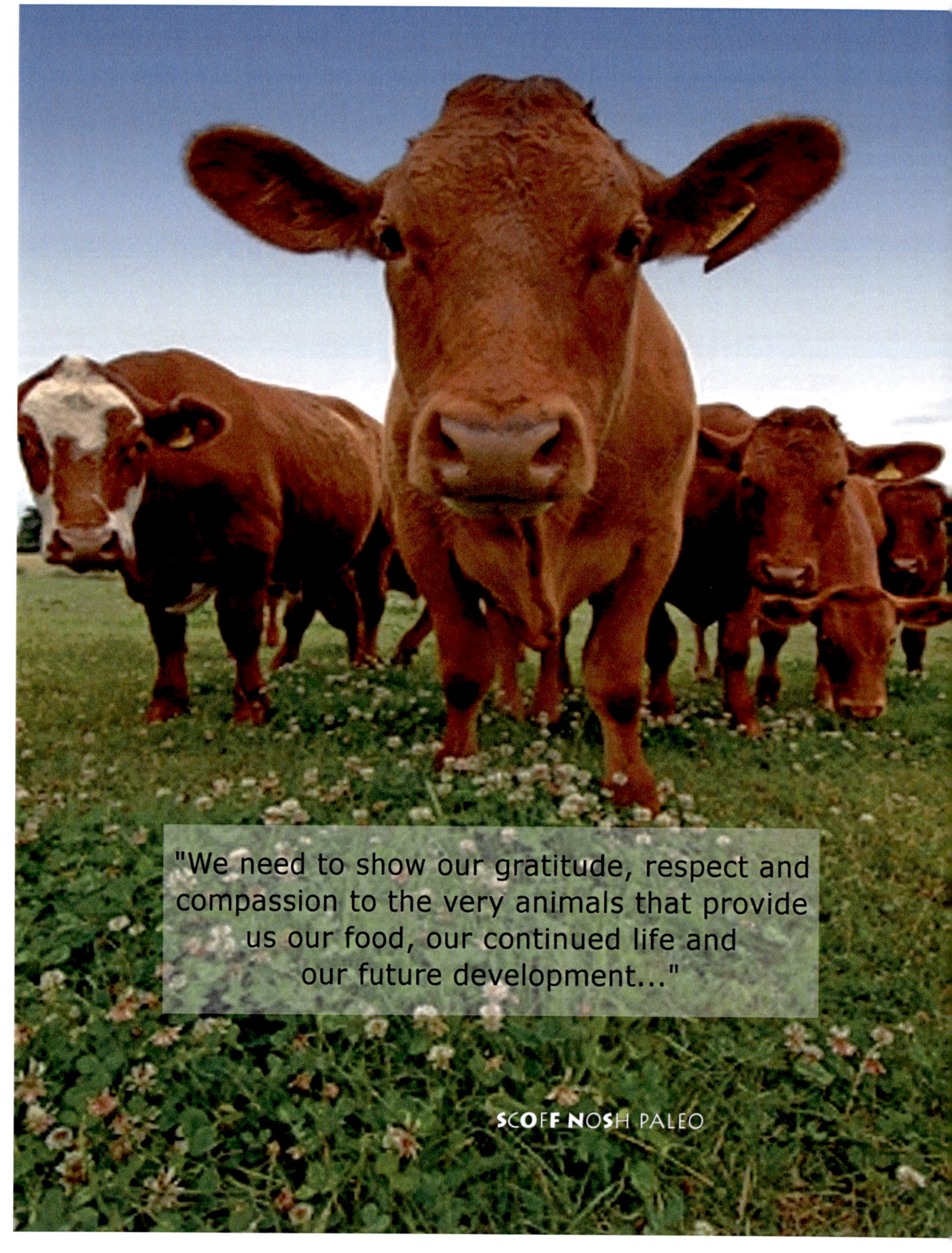

"We need to show our gratitude, respect and compassion to the very animals that provide us our food, our continued life and our future development..."

SCOFF NOSH PALEO

CHAPTER 3

11 HEALTHY BENEFITS OF EATING PALEO.

For most people the fact the Paleo diet delivers the best results is all they need. Improved blood lipids, weight loss, and reduced pain from autoimmunity are proof enough. Many people however are not satisfied with blindly following any recommendations, be they nutrition or exercise related. Some folks like to know WHY they are doing something.

Fortunately, the Paleo diet has stood not only the test of time, but also the rigors of scientific scrutiny.

With a very simple shift we not only remove the foods that are at odds with our health (processed foods, wheat, grains, legumes, and dairy), but we also increase our intake of vitamins, minerals, and antioxidants.

CARDIO VASCULAR DISEASE

According to the CDC, (The Centers for Disease control and Prevention) [5] cardiovascular disease is currently the number one cause of death in the United States. Our Paleolithic ancestors and studied hunter-gatherers showed virtually no heart attack or stroke while eating their ancestral diets. The references below will explore these facts to better help you understand the heart-healthy benefits of a Paleo diet.

AUTO-IMMUNITY

This is a process in which your immune system attacks your own body. Normally our immune system protects us from all bacterial, viral, and parasitic infections. The immune system identifies a foreign invader, attacks it, and then all being well clears the infection.

In auto-immunity, a similar process occurs in that an *individual's* own tissue is confused as something foreign and the immune system attacks this "mislabelled" tissue. Common forms of autoimmunity include Multiple Sclerosis, Rheumatoid Arthritis, Lupus, and Vitiligo, naming just a few of auto-immune diseases.

Elements of auto-immunity are likely at play in conditions as seemingly unrelated as schizophrenia, infertility, and various forms of cancer.

1. CUTS OUT THE CRAVING OF JUNK FOOD

No more frozen pizza or picking up fast food on the way home, or sitting in front of the TV with a bag of cheesies. With Paleo out goes the junk food, this alone means that you're improving your wellbeing, and only spending your money on food that benefits your health.

It's also great for your food budget as these items can sometimes be pricey. Now you can spend these savings on organic meats and vegetables and you'll be doing your health and lifestyle a huge service.

2. BALANCES BLOOD GLUCOSE LEVELS

Largely as you're avoiding refined sugar, it's easier to avoid the spikes in your blood glucose levels, and helps you avoid the sugar crashes and the feelings of fatigue you sometimes get.

If you're diabetic, you may want to check with your doctor to see if they approve of this diet plan. However, if you're simply trying to avoid getting diabetes this will be a better diet choice. Even, if you're not concerned about diabetes and just want to feel better or lose weight, monitoring your blood sugar levels is a great way to do this.

3. MAKES YOU LEANER

Because this diet plan relies on consuming meat as part of your diet you'll be getting a fair amount of protein to give you energy and feed your muscles. This helps to promote a leaner physique, and can help with muscle growth.

When you consider the physique of Stone Age man, they were lean and this sort of efficient physique still helps out today in our modern world. With a leaner body structure you will also be able to better handle life's challenges, including the stresses that occur with your busy 21st century lifestyle.

4. AVOIDS WHEAT AND GLUTEN

You will be automatically cutting out wheat products, which in turn gets rid of the gluten, so in essence, you're following a gluten-free diet at the same time. There is so much evidence suggesting that gluten is problematic both for the digestive system and for rapid weight gain, even for those that don't have Celiac disease, or do not have sensitivity to gluten. I Strongly recommend this read, **WHEAT BELLY** by **Davis MD**, **William**, if you want to look at this topic further. Consuming wheat and Gluten have shown to contribute to larger midsections and sluggish digestion, you immediately improve your body makeup and start to feel better all around.

5. No Calorie Counting Required

Unlike traditional dieting where you are watching points, or counting how many carbs or calories you have in a day, the Paleo diet is intrinsically simple and easy to follow. Remember this diet is what we are genetically designed to eat.

There are no rules or limitations on how much you can have each day. This makes it fun and easy to stick to the plan. By not having to limit yourself, you don't get your brain revolting against you and rejecting the plan resulting in what is know as 'self sabotage'. You're able to simply eat like a human should eat, and how we were designed genetically.

6. Prevents Diseases

By following the Paleo diet you are automatically eating more anti-inflammatory foods, and cutting out many foods that are known to cause inflammation. You are also eating more foods that contain antioxidants and phytonutrients that are always making the news because of scientific evidence that shows them helping to prevent cancers, as well as heart disease.

You're also naturally avoiding a lot of the culprits responsible for disease and illness, like fast food and junk food, so you get a more natural version of yourself and open the doors for healing your whole body and a greater well-being.

7. Helps You Sleep Better

Sleep is so vital, especially in our modern day busy schedules. Simply by cutting out all the chemicals and additives in the typical food sources you'll find that your body naturally gets tired at night. After all, your Body should, and we should listen and act for our greater health and wellness.

Simply put, this is the natural release of serotonin that your brain releases as a signal that it's time to sleep. This would normally be heavily suppressed by a cocktail of chemicals and caffeine in our foods and beverages. When you start to feel sleepy, you should sleep. You might find that you're getting tired earlier at night and that you feel energized and ready to wake up earlier in the morning. This is your body getting in tune with the circadian rhythm, (This is any biological process that displays an endogenous, entrainable oscillation of about 24 hours), *you're now living on natural instinct not chemicals, just like prehistoric man.*

8. Avoids Heavily Processed Foods

This single benefit will have a huge long lasting effect on your health, wellness, as well as make you look younger and feel healthier.

When you cut out processed foods you're cutting out many synthetic chemicals that have just come about in the last 50 years, your genome (your bodies DNA) having developed over 2.6 million years is massively struggling to deal with.

You may be surprised by how many foods get the no-go because of the processing involved, and how much you used to rely on these foods on a day-to-day basis. Some of you may have a hard time giving up dairy products, 'believe me, we were not designed to digest lactose' or products that come out of packets.

There may be a period of both physical and psychological adjustment. Just remember your reading this book because you don't feel right, your fatigued, tired, sluggish, suffering ill health, bloating or digestion issues or have excess weight. So use this as your leveller to make the change. It is a lot easier to undo than you think, *we can't honestly believe after 2.6 million years, our diet wasn't going to return as human nature intended.*

9. Gives You Increased Energy

When you consume a paleo diet in the right way, you're getting well-balanced meals with a protein, carb, and vegetable, and you're getting it from all healthy natural sources.

This is the way to feel more energized and at the top of your game without having to resort to energy drinks, caffeinated beverages, and other means to get you through the day.

Unlike other diets that rely on reduced amount of calories, the Paleo diet allows you to eat until you are satisfied. You should also eat when you feel hungry, so you don't run the risk of running low on fuel when you really need it. This sounds too good to be true...

10. Detox Your Body Naturally

Eating paleo stops you eating the trans fats, MSG, caffeine, refined sugar, gluten, and more. You are giving your body a permanent vacation. By getting more antioxidants from the fruit you'll be eating, and more phytonutrients and fibre from the vegetables you'll be purging your body of built-up waste and accumulation.

Overall eating this diet provides a detoxifying effect to the body, many followers of the paleo diet report feeling lighter and more clear headed after several weeks. The nice thing about it is that it doesn't involve going to extremes like fasting. You get to eat meals like normal, so it's a very smart way of a full detox.

11. Effortless Weight Loss and health

If you do nothing else but start to eat Paleo many will notice the excess weight will disappear. This is because in addition to eating a meal that is more natural, you're cutting out many foods that are processed and unnatural.

When you stop worrying about having to lose weight and temptations and feelings of dread about the foods you're eating, you'll start to see food as fun again, especially as its healthy too. You are now in a total win-win situation.

Do the things that make you happier,
smarter and healthier. ~ Unknown

CHAPTER 4

UNDERSTANDING PALEO NUTRITION.

The Paleo diet is about eating healthy fats and proteins, nutrients and phytonutrients that your body can interpret and process naturally without having to store excess fat. This food is used as fuel for your body and to maintain a healthy metabolism.

Man has discovered how to put sugar and fat in processed food. This is a deadly combination and causing an epidemic of ill health that increases year on year.

Saturated fat consumed by its self the body can deal with, put sugar and fat in processed food THEN this combination is lethal. This does not apply to any other natural food know to man.

THE SIMPLE BUILDING BLOCKS OF A HEALTHY PALEO DIET

LEAN PROTEINS

Lean proteins support strong muscles, healthy bones and optimal immune function. Protein also makes you feel satisfied between meals, giving you your required energy.

FRUITS AND VEGETABLES

Fruits and vegetables are rich in antioxidants, vitamins, minerals and phytonutrients that have been shown to decrease the likelihood of developing a number of degenerative diseases including cancer, diabetes and even neurological decline.

HEALTHY FATS FROM NUTS, SEEDS, AVOCADOS, OLIVE OIL, FISH OIL AND GRASS-FED MEAT.

Saturated fat has been identified as being bad for your health by the health authorities and the media.

Are the current recommendations for VERY low saturated fat intake justified?

How much saturated fat and what types of fats, if any should we eat?

In the absence of historical and scientific data these questions are impossible to answer.

One of the greatest deviations away from our ancestral diet is the amount and types of fat found in modern grain fed animals vs. the amounts and types of fats found in grass fed or wild meat, fowl and fish.

What we have observed is that wild meat is remarkably lean, and has relatively low amounts of saturated fats, while supplying significant amounts of beneficial omega-3 fats such as EPA and DHA.

Analysing the complete fatty acid profile from several species of wild deer and elk. The take home message is that free-range grass fed meat is far healthier than conventional meat for reducing diet-related chronic disease.

Omega-3 and omega-6 fatty acids have opposing functions; yet, both improve your health when they are consumed appropriately.

The **ratio** of these two fatty acids proves fundamental in their health benefits.

Omega-3 and omega-6 are types of essential fatty acids, fatty acids that our bodies cannot make on their own, so we do have to obtain them from our diet. Both are polyunsaturated fatty acids and they differ from each other in their chemical structure. Omega-6 fatty acid increases your blood pressure and inflammatory reactions while omega-3 fatty acids oppose these reactions. Omega-3 fatty acids' double-bond structure makes them essential for building cell walls and developing brain tissue.

Did you know that 90% of us are deficient in them?

Nutrition experts say a healthy ratio of omega-6 to omega-3 in a diet ranges between 1:1-4:1, with an average of 3:1 being optimum for many people. The World Health Organization recommends an omega-6 fatty acid intake of 5-8% of energy and an omega-3 fatty acid intake of 1-2% of energy. In 2002, The Food and Nutrition Board of the U.S. Institute of Medicine established adequate intake (AI) levels for omega-6 and omega-3 fatty acids as follows:

- The AI for men is 14-17 grams (17 for up to 50 years old) of omega-6, and 1.6 grams of omega-3 daily.
- The AI for women is 11-12 grams (12 for up to 50 years old) of omega-6, and

1.1 grams of omega 3 daily.

Today, our western diet has a ratio of up to 30 or more times the amount of omega-6 than omega-3. That's closer to a **10:1 ratio,** and a cause for concern as an excessive intake of either fat supplement can cause harm. Omega-3 fats can contribute to prolonged bleeding and suppression of the immune system. Omega-6 fats can lead to gastrointestinal upset and more.

This dietary imbalance may explain the rise of many diseases as asthma, coronary heart disease, many forms of cancer, autoimmunity and neurodegenerative diseases, all of which are believed to stem from inflammation in the body. The imbalance between omega-3 and omega-6 fatty acids may also contribute to obesity, alcoholism, hyperactivity, depression, manic depression, memory loss, impaired night vision, anxiety, insomnia, dementia, Multiple Sclerosis, Alzheimer's, Parkinson's, ADD, ADHD, dyslexia, schizophrenia, stress induced hostility and even a tendency toward violence.

To avoid this long list of undesirable conditions, what should we eat to strike the right balance?

Employ the Principle of Substitution: Instead of trying to adopt an entirely new diet, use substitution to make gradual improvements. Identify foods that have poor nutritional value and replace them with better ones, especially those with a healthier omega 3 to omega 6 balance. On of the single most effective thing you can do to get your omega balance is to avoid vegetable oils high in omega-6 such as soybean, corn and safflower, and all the processed foods that contain them. A food such as corn oil can be as skewed as 50:1. Meat, poultry, pork and eggs are also sources of omega-6.

Focus on adding more sources of omega-3 to balance out the excess of omega-6 that you're most likely already getting. Some of the most easily digestible forms of omega-3s are found in fatty fish such as salmon, cod and mackerel, but vegetarian diets rich in certain kinds of vegetables, microalgae, nuts and oils can provide the full range of necessary omega-3s.

ESSENTIAL AND NONESSENTIAL AMINO ACIDS FOR HUMANS.

Dietary protein is the main source of amino acids. Amino acids can also be used as fuel, but usually more important roles for them are as building blocks for proteins, and as a source of carbon and nitrogen for biosynthesis of other bio-chemicals.

In the process of our digestion, proteins are broken down into free amino acids in the gastrointestinal tract. They are then absorbed and pass into the circulation, and are transported to the liver, where the NH2 groups are removed by transamination. The resulting alpha-keto acid is then used as fuel, or as a biosynthetic intermediate.

The difference is that amino acids are not stored in the body like fats or carbohydrate; there are no specialized cells in the body to maintain a reservoir. Of course, amino acids are present in structural proteins, enzymes, transport proteins, etc. Some of these proteins (notably serum albumin) can be degraded under conditions of fasting or starvation, to release free amino acids.

Adult humans are unable to synthesize all twenty amino acids needed for protein synthesis; those which cannot be synthesized and which must then be acquired via the diet are referred to as the ESSENTIAL AMINO ACIDS. The ten that the body can self synthesize are known as nonessential.

THE TEN NON ESSENTIAL
AMINO ACIDS FOR ADULTS ARE:-

Phenylalanine, Aline, Tryptophan, Threonine, Isoleucine, Methionine, Histidine

Arginine, Leucine, Lysine

Dietary intake of amino acids is typically not balanced to exactly match the body's demands for various amino acids. The amino acids taken via our diet must be chemically modified and rearranged to provide adequate levels of all the amino acids our body's need.

There are a large number of pathways in the body for balancing the pool of amino acids, both for synthesis and for degradation.

The number of enzymes involved creates a great potential for genetic diseases. Furthermore, disruption (by mutation of just one enzyme) in the metabolism of only one amino acid can have profound consequences for growth and development; some of the genetic diseases are fatal.

Foods with amino acids are the building blocks of protein. That means they are responsible for strength, repair and rebuilding inside your body. Your tissues, your cells, your enzymes and your brain, all get their nourishment and protection from your body's amino acids.

DO I NEED AMINO ACIDS DAILY.
Amino acids make up 75% of the human body, minus water, they are vital to every part of our human function. One of the most talked about properties of amino acids is how they can assist in muscle building and maintenance.

You have probably heard or seen amino acids boasted as the key ingredients in many body building supplements, though the degree of success they achieve in that form is still debatable.

Careful attention to amino acids isn't just for people wanting to build muscle. Different studies have linked amino acid balances with fighting everything from depression to Fibromyalgia.

However You Can't Store Amino Acids.

The problem with amino acids is that they deteriorate with time. Your body does have the ability to store extra starch and protein as fat, to enable us to use it later.

However, Amino acids are not stored <u>they are replaced</u>. There are upwards of twenty different kinds of amino acids that form proteins. Some of these the body makes. The ones it cannot make are called the essential amino acids. You must get these from your regular consumption of food.

THE BEST FOODS FOR OUR ESSENTIAL AMINO ACIDS.

Studies have shown that the best way to get all our essential amino acids, acids not made by your body, is to eat animal protein.

Yes, beef, bison, pork, wild boar, offal, game meat, fish, seafood, poultry and eggs all provide us delicious and superior animal protein your body needs.

Scientists discovered that approximately 1 million years ago our ancestors discovered fire [6] and started to include more animal foods into their diet. This greatly influenced human brain evolution and our brain development began.

We wouldn't be who we are today if we hadn't started including more meat in our diet. By eating less plant foods, our gut decreased in size, allowing in return more energy for the development of our brain.

This evolution would probably not have been possible on a vegetarian diet, let alone a vegan diet. Proteins from animal food are high-quality complete proteins that contain all the essential amino acids your body requires.

Vegetable proteins, from legumes, soy and grains, are incomplete and lack some of the essential amino acids.

Amino acids from protein are the building blocks necessary to build muscles, synthesize the DNA and cells in your body, nourish the cell lining of your intestines and are involved in making enzymes, hormones, proteins fighting for your immune system and proteins that transport vitamins, minerals, cholesterol, fat and other important nutrients inside your body.

If some amino acids are not present in your diet in the right proportions, these functions cannot be accomplished.

What are the Best Animal Protein choices in the Paleo diet?

Grass-fed, grass-finished, pastured, free-range… the terminology can sometimes be complicated especially with the different labelling regulations. One method is to question your supplier, meat can be advertised as NATURAL with few restrictions, but GRASS FED, ORGANIC and CERTIFIED ORGANIC have strict government guidelines and are a safe option.

Why you should try and eat pastured, grass-fed and free-range meat. Stay away from food produced in factory farming conditions this is where animals are confined in cages under unethical conditions and force-fed atrocious quantities of grains, soy and "by-product feedstuff" to make them grow and fatten up as quickly as possible so they can be butchered and sold. No considerations are given to the animals and the environment.

This is why many people go vegetarian. Fortunately these are not the only option!

You can select meat from animals that were treated humanely and grass fed let out to pasture on fields. You can go to your farmers market or find a farm in your area.

Remember that every time you encourage a local farmer and/or buy grass-fed, pastured meat and eggs, you are voting with your money! … and eating less chemicals, hormones and steroids.

My hope is that the more demand there is for high-quality and sustainable foods, as advocated by the Paleo diet, the more widely available and affordable they will become.

Protein is an essential macronutrient that supports almost every type of cell in your body. While it's important to get enough high-quality animal protein, humans were never designed to use it as our main energy source.

If you're new to Paleo, it's especially important to remember that fat, not protein, should make up the bulk of your calories: there's no such thing as "low-fat Paleo." All the calculations about percentages and grams per pound of body weight can be fascinating, but they seem overwhelming, well here's no need to spend time and energy worrying about them.

Simply eating a variety of fatty meats as part of a well-balanced diet should keep most people within a healthy range of protein consumption without needing to pull out the calculator.

IS THE PALEO DIET A HIGH FAT DIET?

Although the macronutrient ratio may vary depending on your personal goals and dietary needs, the Paleo diet tends to be lower in carbs, moderate in protein and high in fat compared to the standard Western diet. This is of course after you cut out all grains, flours, dairy and sugars from your diet, you need to make sure you get adequate energy and fat is your solution!

HOW BADLY HAVE WE BEEN ADVISED?

Most of us are scared of fat and its years of being brain washed to eat low fat food, and even drink low fat milk.

The low-fat message is so ingrained in most of our heads that it may be difficult to believe it at first…

However there is real good science to back up the safety of consuming a higher-fat diet.

A large meta-analysis regrouping 21 studies involving nearly 350,000 subjects followed for 23 years showed that there was absolutely no relationship between cardiovascular diseases and saturated fat intake. These results were published in the January 2010 issue of the American Journal of Clinical Nutrition. [7]

Also many studies clearly show that a high fat intake, in the context of a lower carb diet, is beneficial in terms of, controlling appetite and weight, reducing triglycerides, blood pressure and inflammation, elevating HDL cholesterol levels, and increasing LDL particle size, making them less atherogenic (large, fluffy LDL particles that are less likely to stick to your arteries compared to the small and dense LDL particles often associated with high-carb, low-fat diets).

So what does cause our bad health?

If fat and cholesterol don't cause us health issue like metabolic syndrome, then what does?

Most likely, elevated blood sugar levels, trans fats and easily oxidized and unstable omega-6 fatty acids found in our processed GM foods. This contributes towards inflammation, now thought to be the root cause of many of today's chronic diseases.

Eating fat won't make you fat! For at least 4 decades, nutrition and health surveys show that Americans have gradually decreased their fat intake by choosing low-fat products, avoiding red meat and butter and replacing their fat with more carbohydrates, mainly from grains and sugars.

The result of this low-fat and high-carb diet = Obesity, Hypertension and Type 2 Diabetes with current rates at their highest in history of man… So clearly, this dietary advice is not working… You think!!

It is time to re-evaluate the current dietary guidelines and start exploring alternatives to stop this ill health epidemic, as suggested by the Nutrition & Metabolism Society,[8] an independent non-profit health organization providing research, information and education in the application of fundamental science to nutrition.

The higher fat content of the Paleo diet can help you feel more satisfied and less hungry so you can easily reach your healthy body weight without starving yourself.

Understanding that animal saturated fats are not the evil the government health associations want you to believe they are.

Health professionals and so-called nutrition experts are NOT aware that about half of the fat found in meat, chicken skin and even bacon is actually "heart-healthy" monounsaturated fat!

You can research any reliable nutrition database and find that foods that are vilified because of their saturated fats often contain just as much unsaturated fats.

Here are a few examples:

- 44% of the fat in rendered chicken fat or chicken skin is monounsaturated and 21 % is polyunsaturated,
- 48% of the fat in duck fat is monounsaturated and 12% is polyunsaturated,
- 45 and 60% of the fat in a steak is unsaturated,
- 50 to 55% of the fat in pork is unsaturated,
- 48 to 50% of the fat in bacon and lard is monounsaturated and 10% is polyunsaturated, and
- 40% of the fat in butter is monounsaturated.

Foods with a higher saturated fat and lower polyunsaturated fat content are more stable and less susceptible to oxidation. For example, tallow, lard, coconut oil, ghee and duck fat are suitable for cooking your meat and vegetables, while extra virgin olive oil, avocado oil and macadamia oil should be reserved for cold use only (to drizzle over your food or prepare a homemade salad dressing or mayonnaise to accompany your meals). Using the later at high temperatures causes oxidation.

WHY YOU SHOULD NOT COOK WITH OLIVE OIL!

Olive oil is one of the best sources of the Omega oils that YOU NEED for a healthy nervous system and cardiovascular system...**HOWEVER** those amazing BENEFITS ARE ALMOST COMPLETELY DESTROYED once you heat the oil! That's right, the process of heating oils can cause the fats to become carcinogenic; which means causes **CANCER!** Heating causes enzymes to be destroyed, proteins are denatured, fats become carcinogenic, carbohydrates (sugars) become caramelized, vitamins and minerals become less available, and water is eliminated.

My Paleo cooking depends on coconut oil Coconut oil is 92% saturated fat which makes it really stable under heat and solid at room temperature. I buy the organic virgin coconut oil, it leaves a great yet subtle coconut taste and smell to your dishes. Amazing with seafood's...

CHAPTER 5

OPTIMIZING YOUR DIGESTION.

I seriously contemplated about including this chapter in my book but read on and you will see the importance, you won't be disappointed!

One of the best-kept secrets of medicine is the role of the digestive tract and its relationship to our immune system. The so called Leaky Gut Syndrome; the fact that there's a lot of immune cells in the digestive tract called the Galt system, approximately 70 % of all our immune cells are in the digestive tract.

The role of the intestinal tract in keeping us well is a new and enormous topic that very few endocrinologists know anything about. Proof... about ten to fifteen years ago, they didn't even know what a probiotic was!

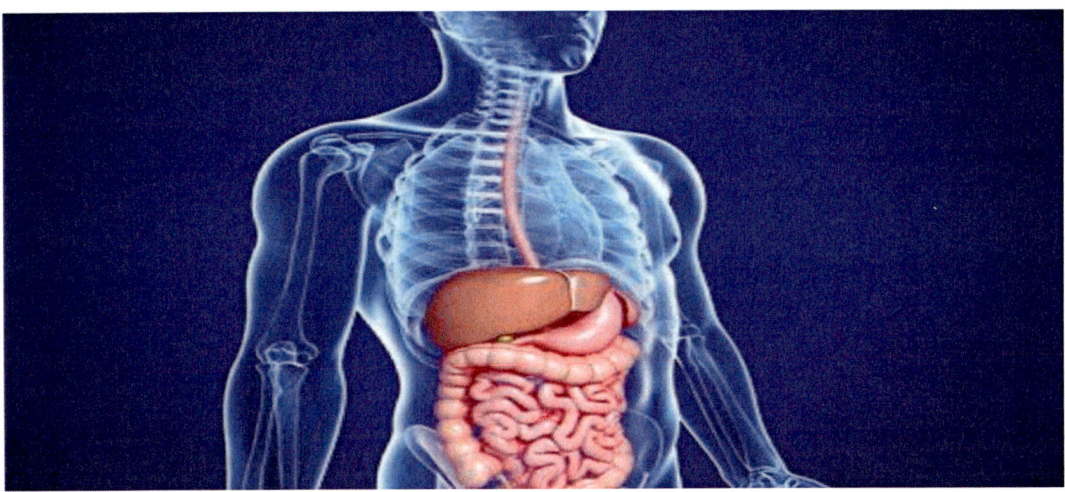

Your digestive tract is 25-35 foot long, it runs from our mouth to your... bum-bum ☺. It is the protective barrier, protecting the rest of our body from the outside environment that consists of foreign invaders such as chemicals, undigested food, toxins and pathogens.

It compromises about 70% of our entire immune system. If we suffer from poor or compromised digestion this actually directly affects your entire immunity and overall health. A healthy gut is indeed a very healthy immune system!

As you know I suffered with digestion issue for years including, IBS, swelling and bloating. Most was linked to my lactose intolerance and heavy consumption of processed foods.

Our digestive system is responsible for breaking down our food into tiny particles that our cells can use for supplies of energy, maintenance and repair.

In order for us to properly function and live, we need our digestive system to digest our food then assimilate it (get it to the right places) and then eliminate what needs to be eliminated (toxins, pathogens, etc.)

When our digestion system works properly, it keeps the good stuff in and gets the bad stuff out. How well our bodies can do this will play a key role in how we feel, our ability to prevent disease, our ability to heal our bodies, and overall impact to our health and longevity.

I'm a firm believer in still doing what we can in order to optimize our digestion. You need to keep in mind that you can be consuming all the best foods for your body…eating whole, quality, organic, pasture-raised and grass-fed foods…but if you can't break it down well and assimilate it, you will not reap the full health benefits from your digestion.

HERE ARE SOME METHODS YOU CAN USE TO OPTIMIZE YOUR DIGESTION?

1) CHEW your food (and your liquids) !!!

YES, an American named Horace Fletcher brought out a simple remedy he called the chew - chew diet. This comprised of eating what you wanted but chewing everything 32 times. This worked extremely well for Fletcher who shed more than 40lbs after four months. It also caught on across the Atlantic in England where it's reported the Victorian's adopted this and dinners were held called 'munching parties'.

This is hard to do but the lesson here is your digestion begins in your mouth. Enzymes are secreted by your salivary glands to help you break down your foods, this is especially true for starches. The physical process of chewing with your teeth also breaks down the food in preparation for the stomach.

2) Eat until you are 80% full. This allows enough space for the digestive juices to fully breakdown food. A good analogy of this I picked up, is explained here:- Think of a furnace ...if you filled the furnace full of wood and then tried to light it you wouldn't create a very good fire because there is not enough space for oxygen to help keep the flames going. In the same way if you fill your stomach full of food then you will not create enough space to ignite your digestive fire.

The following methods are achieved by simply following the Paleo Diet.

3) This is the MOST IMPORTANT try and avoid any processed foods, refined / artificial sugar, acidic foods, fried foods, grain and breads. Your body does not digest preservatives, chemical, wheat, artificial sweeteners etc. easily and not without a detrimental affect on your health.

4) ELIMINATE dairy, grains and legumes. Many people with compromised digestion will need to avoid these foods entirely and it is recommended to do so, at least initially. Some are able to add in raw dairy products (especially fermented dairy) and do quite well with it. As you know 65% of the world population cannot digest the lactose in milk or suffer difficulty in doing so.

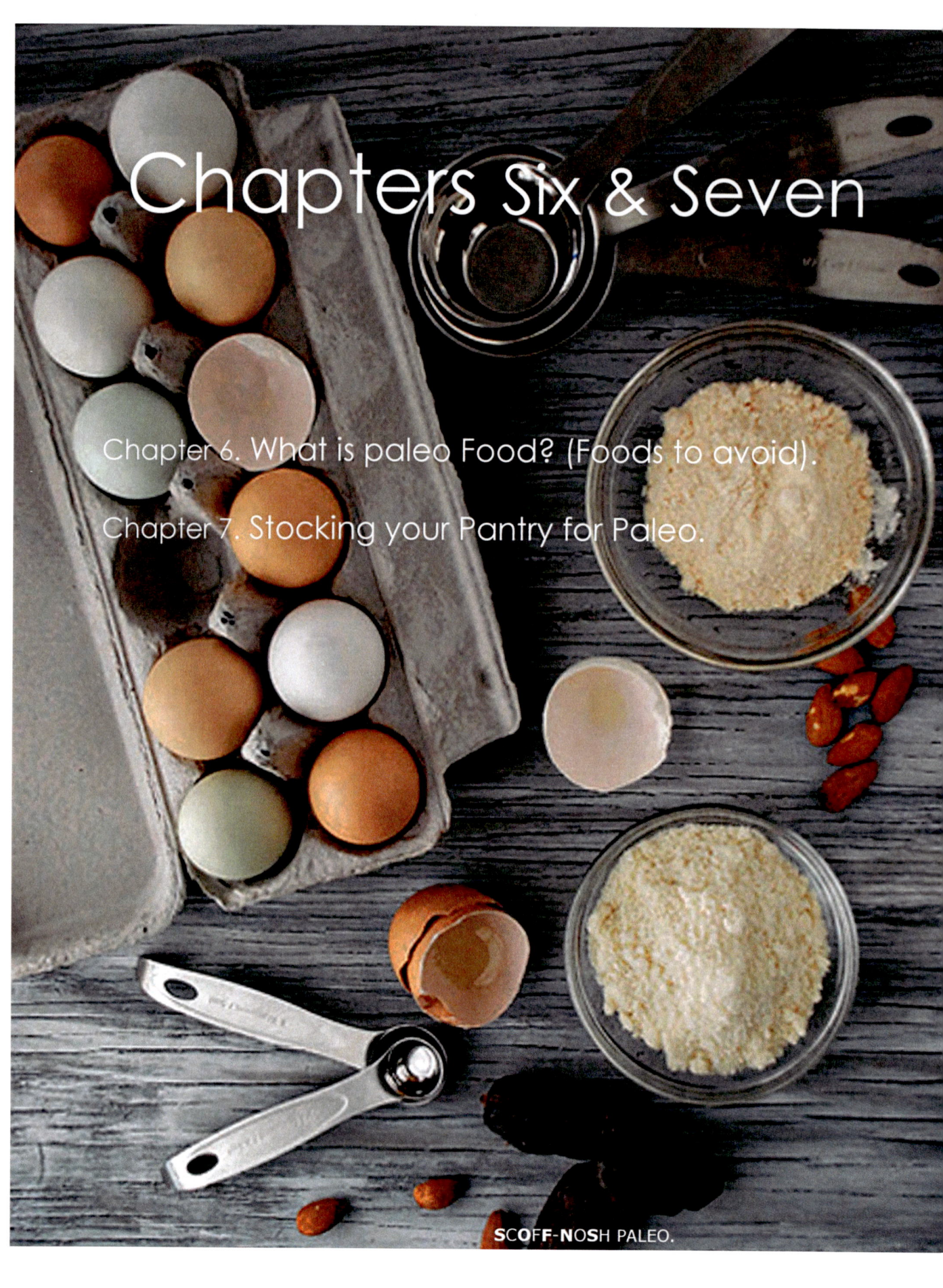

Chapters Six & Seven

SCOFF-NOSH PALEO.

CHAPTER 6

WHAT IS PALEO FOOD? (FOODS TO AVOID)

The following list is my comprehensive paleo diet food list. In this chapter you will find a list of paleo meats, vegetables, fruits, nuts, seeds and oils that are allowed on the paleo diet.

I hope to give you a solid foundation of the paleo diet food list, but I also hope to get your taste buds tingling with the list of ingredients and then we have the amazing recipes.

I have broken this list down into the specific food groups so you can see what types of meats, vegetables, fruits, nuts or fats are on the paleo diet. At the end of the list you will also find a list of foods that are NOT allowed in the Paleo diet.

PALEO DIET FOOD LIST ALLOWED:

PALEO MEATS | PALEO VEGETABLES | PALEO DIET FRUITS

PALEO OILS/FATS | PALEO NUTS |

PALEO DIET FOODS NOT Allowed:

DAIRY | SOFT DRINKS | FRUIT JUICES | LEGUMES | GRAINS | FATTY MEATS | SALTY FOODS | STARCHY VEGETABLES | PROCESSED SNACKS | ENERGY DRINKS | SWEETS

PALEO DIET FOOD LIST ALLOWED:
PALEO MEATS

I have included the list of the Paleo meats allowed in the paleo diet. I recommend where you can to try and eat pasture raised, grass fed meats. NO GRAIN FED, HORMONE AND STEROID RAISED MEAT.

It goes without saying that you should stay away from highly processed meats and meats that are high in fat (fast food burgers, tinned spam and hot dogs are all low-quality meat).

- Poultry
- Turkey
- Chicken Breast
- Pork Tenderloin
- Pork Chops
- Steak
- Veal
- Bacon
- Pork
- Ground Beef
- Grass Fed Beef
- Chicken Thigh
- Chicken Leg
- Chicken Wings (my favourite with salad!)
- Lamb rack
- Shrimp
- Lobster
- Clams
- Salmon
- Venison Steaks
- Buffalo
- New York Steak
- Bison
- Bison Steaks
- Bison Jerky
- Bison Rib eye

- Bison Sirloin
- Lamb Chops
- Goat
- Elk
- Emu
- Goose
- Rabbit
- Beef Jerky
- Eggs (duck, chicken or goose)
- Wild Boar
- Reindeer
- Turtle
- Ostrich
- Pheasant
- Quail

PALEO DIET FISH.

My favourite source of protein is seafood and then steak. Fish are definitely on the paleo diet and they're full of goodness and also Omega 3. The general rule here is if it swims and has fins, it's definitely on the paleo table.

- Salmon
- Halibut
- Mackerel
- Sardines
- Tuna
- Bass
- Red Snapper
- Sunfish
- Tilapia
- Trout
- Walleye

PALEO DIET SEAFOOD.

We are now in my favourite section, seafood, especially shrimp, mussels and crabmeat. Enjoy these in some amazing recipes with various herbs like chili powder, cayenne pepper and paprika. Read on and discover the range of different seafood you can eat on the paleo diet.

- Mussels
- Crab
- Shrimp
- Clams
- Scallops
- Oysters
- Lobster
- Crawfish
- Crayfish

PALEO DIET VEGETABLES.

Vegetables are an integral part of the paleo diet. Almost all vegetables foods are on the paleo diet table. One thing I will say is you should avoid vegetables with high starch content – such as potatoes, and squashes. These generally tend to have low nutritional value in comparison to the amount of starches, carbs and sugars they contain. While these are not really bad for you, there are better nutrient filled options out there.

- Asparagus
- Avocado
- Artichoke hearts
- Brussels sprouts
- Carrots
- Spinach
- Celery
- Broccoli
- Zucchini
- Cabbage
- Peppers (All Kinds)
- Cauliflower
- Parsley
- Eggplant
- Green Onions

- Butternut Squash*
- Acorn Squash*
- Yam*
- Sweet Potato*
- Beets*

PALEO DIET OILS/FATS.

Contrary to popular belief, fat doesn't make you fat. Carbs do (the standard WESTERN diet has a ton of them!). Natural oils and fats are your body's preferred way of creating energy so it's best to give your body exactly what it's asking for! The following are the best types of paleo oils and fats that you can give your body for additional sustained energy.

- Coconut oil
- Olive oil virgin organic
- Macadamia Oil
- Bacon Fat / Lard
- Avocado Oil
- Grass fed Butter Only
- Ghee
- Duck Fat

PALEO DIET NUTS.

Nuts are paleo ?!? *I go totally against the common trend in the paleo diet here, my advice is to try and limit the quantity of nuts you consume. One of the main principles of the paleo diet is to avoid eating grains and legumes because of the toxins they contain. One of those toxins phytic acid (phytate) is emphasized as one of the biggest offenders.*

What most people aren't told when they start the paleo diet is that nuts are often as high or even higher in phytic acid than GRAINS. In fact, nuts decrease iron absorption even more than WHEAT BREAD. [10]

In the paleo diet we go to great lengths to avoid food toxins yet some people are still eating nuts like crazy.

What is phytic acid and what does it do?

Phytic acid is the storage form of phosphorus found in many plants, it is especially found in the bran or the hull of grains and also in nuts and seeds.

Although herbivores like cows and sheep can digest phytic acid, us humans can't. The phytic acid actually binds to minerals (especially iron and zinc) in food and prevents our bodies from absorbing these minerals. Recent studies show that we absorb approximately 20 % more zinc and 60 % more magnesium from our food when phytic acid is not present in our gut. [11]

The phytic acid interferes with the enzymes that we need to digest our food, this includes pepsin, and this is vital for the breakdown of proteins in our digestion and amylase, which is required for the breakdown of starch.

Phytic acid also inhibits the enzyme trypsin, which is needed for protein digestion in the small intestine. As most people following a paleo diet probably know diets high in phytate acid cause mineral deficiencies, i.e. osteoporosis are common where cereal grains are a staple part of their diet. [12]

- Almonds
- Hazelnuts
- Pecans
- Pine Nuts
- Pumpkin Seeds
- Sunflower Seeds
- Macadamia Nut
- Walnuts
- Cashews

Just in case you were wondering, Peanuts are NOT a nut and NOT Paleo!!!

I personally don't eat many raw nuts, I feel it hugely contradictory to my diet by excluding grains for their negative properties, yet indulging in nuts with the same or higher negative values. I have included in my recipes nuts and now and again in these portions, I don't see any negative impact. I do however limit and sometimes exclude nuts from certain recipes.

PALEO DIET FRUITS.

Being an advocate of The Green Juice Diet mixing fruit with veggies I can confirm that these are an integral part of our diet. What you need to remember is some fruits (even the paleo-approved ones) contain large amounts of fructose, while this is much better than HFCS (high-fructose corn syrup) – it is still sugar.

So if you're looking to lose weight on the paleo diet, you'll want to cut back on the fruit intake and focus more on the vegetables allowed on the paleo diet. You can have 1-3 servings of fruit a day and stay very healthy.

- Avocado
- Apple
- Blackberries
- Bananas*
- Papaya
- Cantaloupe**
- Raspberries
- Peaches**
- Plums
- Mango
- Lychee
- Blueberries
- Grapes
- Lemon
- Strawberries**
- Watermelon**
- Pineapple Guava
- Lime
- Tangerine
- Figs
- Oranges

**Eat high-sugar fruits in moderation. They're great for you, but can be easy to overdo.

*You will notice while starchy foods are good for your energy replacement for paleo diet athletes who are spending long periods of time exercising. As long as you're training, you'll find these are great sources of energy replacements, especially post - workouts. However, if you want to lose weight fast on the paleo diet, you will want to enjoy but limit the quantity of starch and fruit.

So there you have it! This is the comprehensive list of food allowed in the paleo diet. Now lets put these amazing foods together and start enjoying this food...

FOODS NOT ALLOWED ON THE PALEO DIET

So here is the list of foods not allowed on the paleo diet Paleo. By this point you should be comfortable letting go of these foods, after all, no one wants poor health from eating food, do they?

Dairy

- Butter
- Cheese
- Cottage Cheese
- Non fat dairy creamer
- Skim milk
- 2% milk
- Whole milk
- Dairy spreads
- Cream cheese
- Powdered milk
- Yogurt
- Pudding
- Frozen Yogurt
- Ice Milk
- Low fat milk
- Ice cream

Soft drinks

Soft drinks, fizzy pop and coke are jam packed with sugar and high fructose corn syrup and are definitely NOT paleo.

- Coke
- Sprite
- Pepsi
- Mountain Dew… and any other soft drink you can imagine.

Fruit Juices

Fruit juices are very high in sugar (fructose) and will throw your paleo diet off track. Stay away from all these ones.

- Apple Juice
- Orange Juice
- Grape Juice
- Strawberry Juice
- Star fruit Juice
- Mango Juice

Grains

Anything that has a grain in it you should avoid on the paleo diet. YES I DO MEAN ANYTHING.

- Wheat
- Corn, (including corn syrup)
- Cereals
- Bread
- English Muffin
- Toast
- Sandwiches
- Wheat Thins
- Crackers
- Oatmeal
- Cream of Wheat
- High Fructose Corn Syrup
- Pancakes
- Hash Browns
- Beer
- Pasta
- Fettuccini and Lasagne

Legumes

What are legumes? They are simply a dried fruit and are often contained within a shell or a pod. Here is a list of Legumes that are strictly NOT included in Paleo food.

- Black Beans
- Broad Beans
- Fava Beans
- Garbanzo Beans
- Horse Beans
- Kidney Beans
- Lima Beans
- Adzuki Beans
- Navy Beans
- Pinto Beans
- Red Beans
- Green Beans
- String Beans
- Peas
- Black Eyed Peas
- Chickpeas
- Snow peas
- Sugar snap peas
- Peanuts
- Peanut butter
- Miso
- Lentils
- Lupins
- Mesquite
- Soybeans
- All soybean products and its derivatives
- Torfu

Salty Foods

These overly salty foods fall outside the paleo guidelines.

• French Fries
• Ketchup (very high in sugar too)

Snacks

Processed and packaged snacks are definitely NOT paleo.

• Pretzels
• Chips
• Triscuits
• Wheat Thins
• Cookies
• Sun Chips
• Pastries.

Starchy Vegetables

Yes these are still vegetables but you want to stay away from them due to their high starch content.

• Potatoes
• Sweet Potatoes*
• Yucca
• Batata
• Butternut Squash*
• Acorn Squash*
• Yam*
• Beets*

*These are included but in moderation only.

Energy Drinks

Probably the worst product in the world today, bar NONE. I would NEVER advocate anyone EVER to drink these so-called energy drinks. They are highly addictive and on average contain 13, YES, THIRTEEN, teaspoons of refined sugar per drink. They are a huge conflict in terms and should say *"unhealthy addictive sugar rush of energy with a severe energy crash!"*

The sad fact is that these drinks are targeted towards kids.

- Red Bull
- Monster
- Starbucks Refreshers
- Mountain Dew MDX
- Vault
- XS Energy Drink
- 5 Hour Energy

Alcohol

Yes we are now were reaching the sad part, however… remember the 80 – 20 rule we spoke about earlier, this comes in handy here! Nearly all alcohol is not paleo. This includes but isn't limited to:

- Beer
- Whiskey
- Tequila
- Rum
- Vodka
- Alcohol + Mixers

Sweets

Sugar is in almost all refined processed food and should be avoided in the paleo diet. This means cutting out delicious but destructive sweets and sugars that are standard in the Western Diet.
However, raw unrefined natural honey is acceptable.

Snickers, Milky Way, Reese's, Payday, M&Ms, Skittles, Twizzlers, Hershey's, Nestle Crunch, Almond Joy, etc.

Paleo Kitchen Tool Essentials

The Essentials

1. A good **Paleo** recipe Cookbook. **(Good Choice!)**
2. Kitchen scales (measurements are essential)
3. Measuring cups / Jug (Like I said get these right recipes will be amazing)
4. Kitchen sieve
5. Plastic spatular
6. Collection of good quality pyrex bowls
7. Electric or handheld whisk
8. Large wood & Medium plastic chopping board
9. Wooden mixing spoons
10. Chefs kitchen Knifes

Making Life easier & better baking

1. Kitchenaid Food mixer
2. Slow Cooker
3. Non Stick pans and baking trays

SCOFF-NOSH PALEO

CHAPTER 7

STOCKING UP YOUR PALEO PANTRY.

Before you can stock your paleo pantry / larder, one of the first things you should do is remove anything that is "non-paleo". After all, we are human and might be overcome with the urge to eat these foods!

We are all conditioned as a nation to eat convenience foods.

After you remove all of the processed foods, go and restocked your cupboards with your favourite paleo recipe items, herbs, spices and healthy oils and fats, meats, fruits and vegetables

We actually ran our food cupboards down while I was researching my favourite paleo recipes. I wanted to start with making my paleo food-shopping list. The most important meal I found was a good healthy and convenient breakfast and HEALTHY snacks, these were critical!

We started shopping at Farmers Markets and Natural Food stores. However, over the past 2 years the main supermarkets are now becoming aware of consumer changes and trends, they are stocking a good range of foods for the paleo table. We didn't really have to learn new ways to cook, it was using new ingredients and actually flavouring the foods with natural herbs and spices. This was different, however it was also very exciting too!

When everything you eat tastes delicious and makes you feel good, you really don't feel like you are missing out on anything.

There is a short "weaning process" that most people go through when they start out eating paleo. The ultimate goal is to eat organic fruits, vegetables and some nuts as well as grass fed proteins.

There are many paleo recipes that include foods such as nut butters, nut flours, raw honey, etc. These are much healthier options than your regular wheat flours and refined sugars, and they are a good starting point to help you ease into your paleo lifestyle.

So, should you eat paleo desserts or snacks every single day? In short, No, these are treats and should be eaten in moderation, especially if your goal is to lose weight. But if you are craving a cookie, you are much better off eating a cookie made from ground up almonds and raw honey than if you are eating one made with hydrogenated oils and topped with sugar-filled icing.

If you have a family that you are trying to adjust to a paleo lifestyle, recreate the food recipes your family are familiar with, but using paleo ingredients this will make that transition a lot easier.

I truly wanted to start living the paleo lifestyle so I found the paleo transition quite easy.

My advice to you is if your not 100% committed after reading this book, or want to ease yourself into paleo, that's GREAT! Start experimenting with just one or two paleo meals, making the Paleo equivalent to your current favourite meals.

It's a way of testing the water and easing yourself into the diet. It's a huge healthy step in the right direction, so be happy and proud you are making it.

One of the best things when you get going is to put your own take on recipes, or turning your old favourite foods into paleo food. Using herbs and spices and getting the fresh delicious flavours from your food is truly something else. This is when you know you have arrived at the paleo table. I also don't see any harm in starting at 20% paleo and then 30% paleo and so forth until you are up to 80%. Giving your self that 20% margin for error is safe.

If you are at 80% paleo 100% of the time, you are in very good health. You will start to look at food and meal times completely differently.

"One of the best memories I have when we started to eat paleo was our son luca, at the aged 2 years old while we were at the supermarket. He was helping us shop and recognizing the foods we eat he was picking up the zucchini, bananas and apples … what an amazing healthy habit to bring our son up with. I truly know as he grows up he will lead a healthy life and make healthy food choices, normal to him, but healthy food to anyone else. That's priceless and my total motivation to share this diet with everyone else out there... Enjoy your paleo lifestyle with love, health and lots of fun!"

THE 3 BEST PALEO BAKING FLOURS

Following the all-natural, grain free, low glycaemic diet that our ancestors ate means eating cakes, cookies and breads are no longer on the menu…

Thanks to an amazing choice of all natural sweeteners and flour alternatives, this is no longer the case.

The first step we need to take is to look at the type of flour choices you have for paleo baking. Most people believe that cooking with whole grain flour instead of typical refined white flours is healthier. This is not the case, whole grain flours are still high in carbohydrates and score very high on the glycemic index. High glycemic foods cause a rapid spike in your blood sugar and insulin levels. Over a period of time, this causes a whole spectrum of health problems. Elevated blood sugar levels are linked to most chronic diseases. These include diabetes, cancer, heat disease, metabolic syndrome, obesity and MANY MORE health problems.
Insulin has also been called the "fat storage hormone"

THE REALLY GOOD NEWS HERE IS THAT TRULY HEALTHY OPTIONS ARE NOW AVAILABLE.

These flours are truly versatile. They provide a rich buttery taste to all kinds of baked goods from breads to grain free biscuits and muffins to cupcakes.

ALMOND MEAL/FLOUR.

This staple flour can be used to bake everything from fluffy pancakes to cookies and healthy crackers.

"IT IS BEST TO ONLY USE BLANCHED ALMOND FLOUR, THIS CONTAINS NO SKINS AND LEAVES NO UNPLEASANT AFTERTASTE WHEN BAKED".

HAZELNUT AND PECAN FLOUR.

These flours are a little bit richer than the others and are best used in a combination with almond flour this also increases the nutty flavours to your baking. Theses flours are especially good for baking pie crusts and make very tasty cookies.

TIP.

Nut flours do contain healthy fats but they must be stored in airtight containers, away from sunlight and any heat. If possible they do really well refrigerated. When bought in bulk you can easily freeze this flour in airtight bags.

COCONUT FLOUR.

This flour appears to be very light and fluffy textured, it is in fact quite a dense and fibre rich flour. The secret here is a little flour goes a long way. A good guide here is to use one egg for every tablespoon of coconut flour in your baking. Most of the recipes calling for coconut flour actually specify, *"sifted flour"*.

"THIS IS AN IMPORTANT POINT, AS ONE CUP OF COCONUT FLOUR DOES NOT EQUAL ONE CUP OF SIFTED COCONUT FLOUR".

Always sift the flour then measure it, this will prevent your baking becoming excessively dry or dense.

"BREADS MADE WITH COCONUT FLOUR HAVE AMAZING TASTE AND TEXTURE".

CONVERTING COCONUT FLOUR FOR BAKING.

So we can substitute coconut flour for baking in a recipe, however, the replacement is <u>NOT</u> **ONE** for **ONE** for other flours, alot of people make this mistake and have disappointing flat or dense baking results.

Here is a simple conversion to keep your baking results Healthy, light, fluffy, mouth watering and delicious.

1 CUP OF WHEAT, ALMOND, HAZELNUT
& PECAN FLOUR

=

1/3 CUP
OF COCONUT FLOUR

+ INCREASE YOUR EGGS

DOUBLE EGGS

+ INCREASE LIQUIDS

ADD MORE WATER, COCONUT or ALMOND MILK.

YOUR PALEO SHOPPING LIST.

Below are the recommended items you should try to keep on hand (other than your preferred meats, fruits and vegetables). This is some of the items and a few extra we gathered when we began our paleo diet. If you browse the paleo recipes, you will come across most of them. You can review some of the recipes, see what you want to try and get your herbs spices and ingredients from there, in no time you will be fully paleo stocked up with ingredients.

OILS AND FATS.

Virgin olive oil.

I use virgin olive oil in all my dressings and sauces, (where required), However I stick to the coconut oil or animal fats for the higher heat cooking. Olive oil mixed with balsamic vinegar and some spices makes a great sauce for vegetables and proteins as well.

Coconut Oil

Organic, extra-virgin coconut oil is great for high-temperature cooking and baking. There are many studies on the benefits of coconut oil.

Avocado Oil

This is edible oil pressed from the fruit of the avocado. This is used as an ingredient in other dishes and cooking oil too. It is also used for lubrication and in cosmetics where it is valued for its regenerative and moisturizing properties.

Ghee

Ghee is like butter but has almost all of the protein and lactose removed.

SAUCES FLAVOURING.

Coconut Aminos

A soy-free seasoning sauce made from coconut tree sap, which is used as a substitute for soy sauce. I use this frequently.

Fish Sauce

Red Boat is the most paleo of the fish sauces currently available. I don't use this often, but when I do, it adds a much-needed flavour to my cooking.

Balsamic Vinegar

Great on salads or drizzled on vegetables and proteins, balsamic Vinegar will brighten up any dish so make sure to keep some handy. Not all folks agree that vinegar is paleo - so you decide if you want to use it or not.

Apple Cider Vinegar

This is supposed to cure all sorts of things. Again, not everyone agrees that vinegar is paleo so use it only if you think it is right for you.

Raw Honey

Use this in place of sugar to add sweetness. Raw honey will be mostly solid and you just need to warm it up a little to get it to a liquid state.

Sesame Oil

Sesame oil adds flavour to many different things, so it is great to have on hand. This is great in Asian dishes and in salads.

Mustard

Mustard is a great seasoning that adds a kick to any meal. Make sure it is both gluten and dairy free.

Curry paste

Many curry pastes are paleo and make a great meal when combined with coconut milk, sliced vegetables and proteins.

ONE THING THAT'S ABSOLUTELY ESSENTIAL FOR YOUR PALEO KITCHEN

IS A WELL-STOCKED SPICE RACK.

You should aim to have the following spices on hand:
• Sea salt (preferably Pink Himalayan) or Uniodized Sea salt)• Black pepper• Smoked paprika• Chili powder• Basil• Curry• Coriander• Turmeric• Cinnamon• Thyme• Rosemary

HERE IS A LIST OF 25 HERBS TO HAVE IN YOUR KITCHEN & THEIR HEALTHY BENEFITS.

- **Basil:** full of minerals and a natural antioxidant.
- **Black pepper:** anti bacterial, antioxidant and helps to stimulate digestion.
- **Cardamom:** fresh breath.
- **Cayenne pepper:** antibacterial, rich in beta-carotene, pre cursor to vitamin A, reduces pain and helps stimulates metabolism.
- **Chili pepper:** rich in vitamin C, anti-inflammatory and natural antioxidant
- **Cinnamon:** regulates blood sugar levels, powerful antioxidant, regulates cholesterol metabolism and promotes good circulation
- **Clove:** powerful antioxidant, anti-inflammatory and a mild anesthetic.
- **Coriander:** rich in iron and magnesium, prevents gas, prevents urinary infections, regulates blood sugar levels and is a natural detoxifier of heavy metals.
- **Dill:** anti bacterial, antioxidant and contains a lot of iron
- **Fenugreek:** relieves constipation, and said to stimulate muscle growth.
- **Ginger:** antiseptic, calms the stomach, anti-inflammatory and an effective natural remedy for motion sickness
- **Ginkgo biloba:** is one of the longest living tree species in the world. It stimulates the circulation, anti-aging and improves memory.
- **Garlic:** anti bacterial, anti-viral, lowers blood pressure and has natural antibiotic properties
- **Mustard seed:** rich in selenium, omega-3, phosphorus, vitamin B3 and zinc, helps against cancer and is a natural anti-inflammatory.
- **Nutmeg:** anti-inflammatory and helps to regulates sleep
- **Oregano:** anti bacterial, strong antioxidant and useful as preservative.
- **Paprika powder:** anti-inflammatory and a natural antioxidant
- **Parsley:** detoxifies, helps with kidney stones and a natural antispasmodic.

- **Pepper:** contains a lot of capsaicin, (the ingredient that ensures the 'heat'), clears stuffy noses, relieves pain and said to be beneficial for prostate cancer.
- **Rosemary:** keeps the genes young, strengthens the immune system, improves the circulation and stimulates digestion.
- **Sage:** improves the memory, anti-inflammatory and a strong natural antioxidant.
- **Thyme:** antiseptic and a natural anti bacterial.
- **Turmeric:** often called Curcuma, yellow root or curcumine. A very strong antioxidant, it is said have a role in cancer prevention, help with skin infections, anti-inflammatory and relieves arthritis symptoms.

In the Pantry / Larder.

Stock up on canned foods, but you should only you to buy them if you know they are BPA-free. Otherwise, look for the items produced in glass containers. That being said, a well-stocked Paleo-friendly pantry should contain the following:

- Tomatoes (a variety of diced and whole)

- Coconut milk (full fat)

- Tuna, salmon and crab.

- Virgin organic coconut oil.

- Coconut flour. Almond Flour, Hazelnut and pecan Flour.

- Arrowroot flour (An excellent substitute for cornstarch)

- Almond Flour (Also called ground almonds)

- Pecans, almonds, brazil nuts (make sure the are unsalted)

- Vanilla Cocoa powder

In the refrigerator.

Stock your shelves with lots of fresh veggies. On the Paleo plan, you eat fruit sparingly, but you'll be eating as many vegetables as you possibly can. Make sure you have a good variety of frozen and fresh wild-caught fish, red meat, pork and chicken. Always look for pasture-raised and grass fed meats. Keep a couple dozen farm fresh eggs in your fridge, organic free.

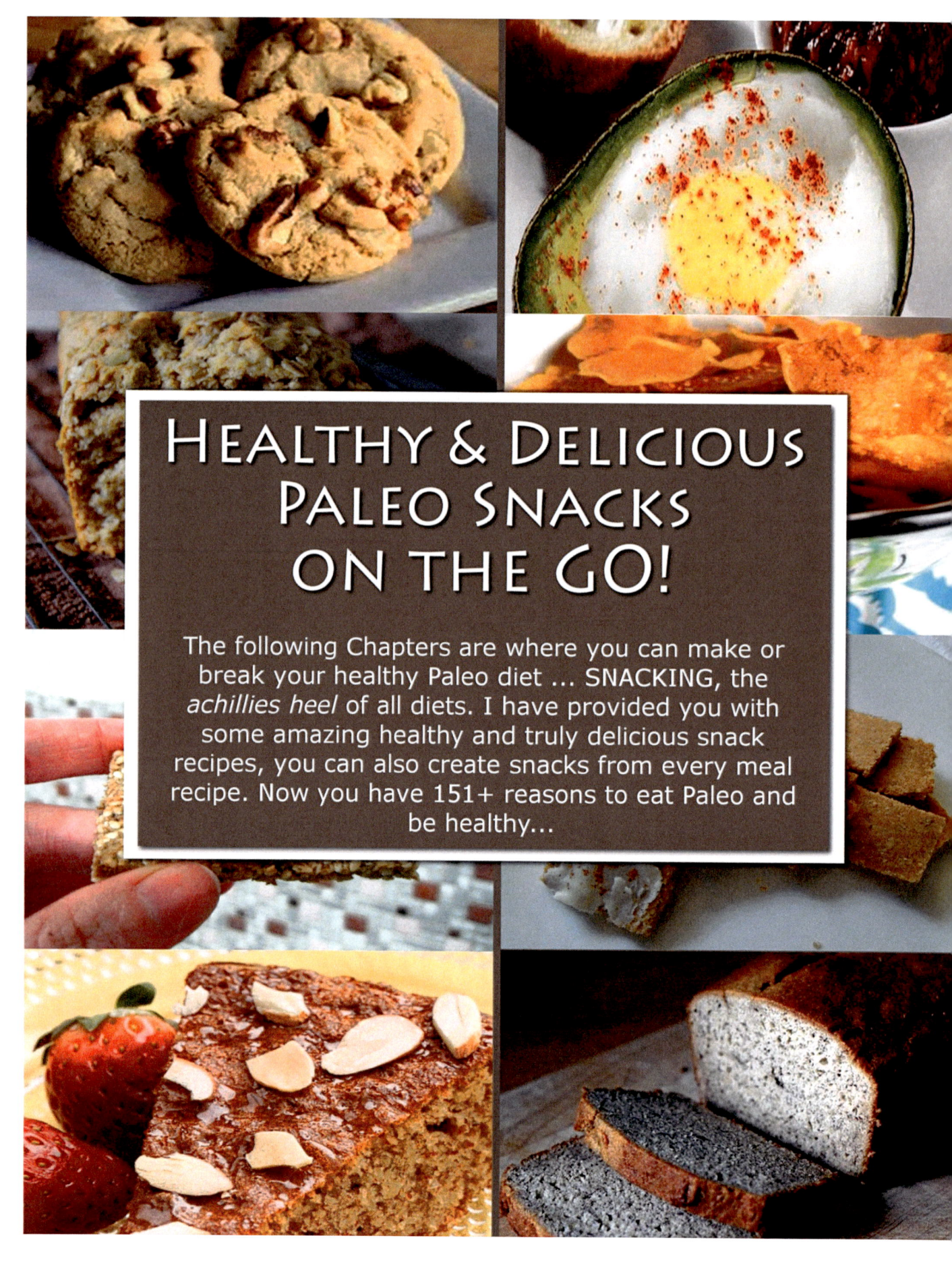

HEALTHY & DELICIOUS PALEO SNACKS ON THE GO!

The following Chapters are where you can make or break your healthy Paleo diet ... SNACKING, the *achillies heel* of all diets. I have provided you with some amazing healthy and truly delicious snack recipes, you can also create snacks from every meal recipe. Now you have 151+ reasons to eat Paleo and be healthy...

CHAPTER 8

PALEO ON THE GO!   HEALTHY SNACKS.

Grain-Free Crackers

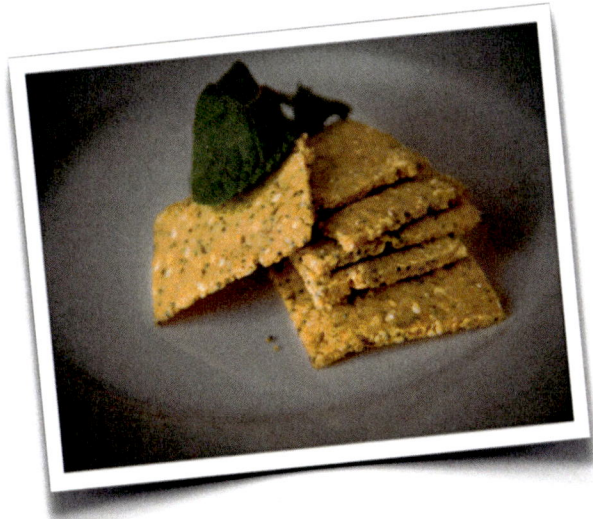

INGREDIENTS
- 1 3/4 cup almond flour
- 1/4 cup combined seeds (I used poppy, sesame, and caraway)
- 1/2 teaspoon sea salt (use coarse if you like the occasional pop of salt)
- dash garlic powder, optional
- 1 Tablespoon melted coconut oil
- 1 egg, well beaten

DIRECTIONS
Preheat oven to 325.

Combine all ingredients and mix / knead well.

Turn out onto a cookie sheet sized piece of parchment paper. Top with another piece of parchment paper and roll out to about 1/8 inch thick. Remove the top sheet of parchment and cut into 1-2 inch squares with a sharp knife.

Bake for 14-20 minutes, or until the crackers are golden brown.

The outside ones may cook first, and it's OK to carefully remove them as they do, then cook the remainder for a few minutes more. Finally cool then store in an airtight container.

Gluten Free Paleo Crackers

These crackers make a great snack and they taste good with any topping. My favourite toppings to put on these crackers are an avocado spread and coconut butter (as seen in this picture).

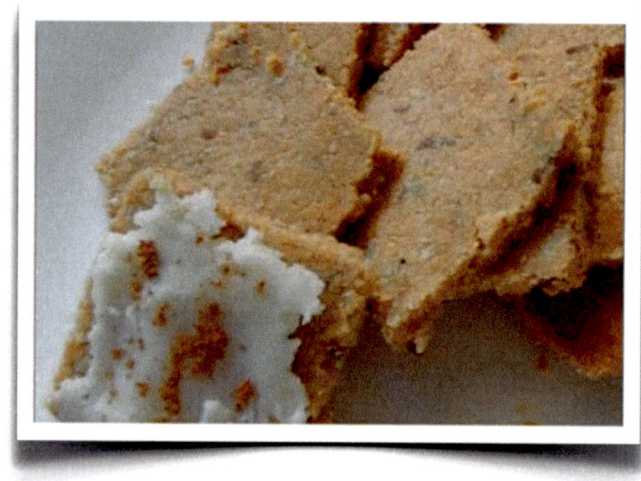

INGREDIENTS

- 1 1/2 cups of almond flour
- 1/4 teaspoon sea salt
- 1 egg
- 1/2 teaspoon olive oil
- 2 tablespoons cinnamon
- 1 1/2 tablespoons flaxseeds

DIRECTIONS

Combine almond flour, sea salt, cinnamon, and flaxseeds in a large bowl.
In a separate bowl, whisk together the egg and olive oil.
Combine the wet and dry ingredients.
Make the dough into a ball. Place on a cookie tray or on parchment paper.
Use a rolling pin to roll out the dough until it reaches 1/16 inch thick.
Cut the dough into 1-inch squares.
Bake at 350° F for 17 to 20 minutes.
Recipe makes approx. 20 crackers.

Gluten-free, Carb-free, Paleo Super Crackers.

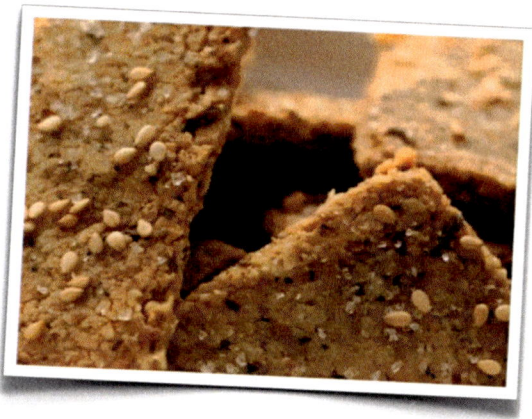

INGREDIENTS

- 2-3 cups almond meal (Make this by grinding almonds in a food processor until fine. Do not to over-blend or you'll have almond butter)
- 1 egg
- 2 tablespoons olive oil, plus more for coating
- 1 teaspoon crushed red pepper
- 1 teaspoon garlic powder
- 1 tablespoon mixed herbs (I used basil, oregano, chives, rosemary and
- parsley)
- sesame seeds for sprinkling (optional)

DIRECTIONS

Preheat oven to 400 degrees. Mix all ingredients thoroughly with your fingers. Divide into four parts and roll out flat on parchment paper with a rolling pin or other cylindrical object Roll out to approx. 1/8 or 1/10 of an inch thick and cut in desired shape with a pizza cutter.

Place individual crackers about one-half-inch apart on a parchment- or tin-foil-lined cookie sheet. Brush the tops of the crackers with olive oil, salt generously and sprinkle with sesame seeds. Bake at 400 degrees for 10-12 minutes, or until crackers are golden brown and crispy.

Coconut Flour Bread

INGREDIENTS

- 6 eggs
- 1/2 cup melted coconut oil
- 1-2 tablespoons honey (optional, I usually leave it out)
- 1/2 teaspoon sea salt
- 3/4 cup coconut flour

DIRECTIONS

Mix all ingredients together and pour into a small oiled loaf pan. Bake at 350 degrees for 40 minutes.

Turn the loaf out and cool completely on a rack before serving.

Coconut and Cinnamon Banana Bread

INGREDIENTS

- 6-8 eggs
- 2 mashed ripe bananas
- 2 teaspoons vanilla
- 5 teaspoons cinnamon
- 1/2 teaspoon salt
- 1/2 cup melted coconut oil
- 1 tablespoons maple syrup or honey
- 1 teaspoon baking powder
- 1/2 cup shredded coconut
- 3/4 cup coconut flour

DIRECTIONS

Preheat oven to 350 degrees F.

Mix all ingredients together until well combined. Pour into 6 mini loaf pans or 12 muffin tins.

Bake for 40-45 minutes (muffins take less time than mini loaves).

Deviled Eggs

INGREDIENTS

- 6 hard-boiled eggs, peeled
- 3 tablespoons of paleo mayonnaise.
- 1/2 teaspoon ground mustard
- 1/8 teaspoon salt
- 1/8 teaspoon cayenne Pepper or
- 1/8 teaspoon black pepper

DIRECTIONS

Cut eggs lengthwise in half. Slip out yolks and mash with fork.
Stir in mayonnaise, mustard, salt and pepper. Fill whites with egg yolk
mixture, heaping it lightly. Cover and refrigerate up to 24 hours.
Cut a very thin slice off the bottom of each egg white before filling to
help the eggs stay in place on the serving plate.

Baked Butternut Squash Chips

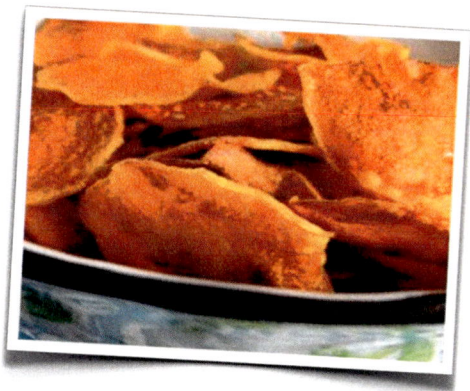

INGREDIENTS

- 1 butternut squash, preferably one with a long, narrow neck
- Spray olive oil
- Pinch of salt to taste
- Special tool required: mandolin

DIRECTIONS

Heat oven to 400 degrees

Set up an ice bowl.

Spray a large baking sheet with olive oil Bring a pot of salted water to boil Cut off the bulb part of the squash and set aside for another use. Peel the skin off the squash and cut crosswise into 3-inch chunks. Using your mandolin cut the squash, crosswise into 1.3mm slices.

Blanch the squash in the boiling water, about two minutes then transfer it to the ice bath to cool. Dry all of the chips with a towel or paper towel and lay them out on the baking sheet. Spray them with olive oil and sprinkle lightly with salt or spices. Set the squash on your oven's middle rack and bake until golden brown and crispy. Keep watching them as some may cook faster than others, even though they are sliced evenly. Season and serve.

Your choice for chips does not end here you can also try Zucchini, banana, carrots etc. ENJOY!

Paleo Cinnamon Apple Muffins

INGREDIENTS

- 1/2 cup almond meal/flour
- 5 large eggs
- 2 medium apples, peeled, cored and chopped
- 2 medium bananas
- 1/2 cup almond oil
- 1 tsp. baking soda
- 2 Tbs. ground cinnamon
- 1/2 cup water
- 1 Tbs. walnut oil

DIRECTIONS

Preheat to 350F. I put apples and bananas in a LARGE bowl and used a potato masher to smooth together. I added everything but the walnut oil and mixed with a spatula. Drop in mixture about 3/4 of the way. Bake for 15 minutes and check and bake for another 5 minutes if required.

Makes 19 muffins. Let them cool before removing from muffin tin. Refrigerate and they will last for approximately 5 days.

Tip:- if you have empty muffin cups in your tray, fill the empty ones with water while baking to ensure even oven temperature! Number of Servings: Many... ENJOY!

....

Almond & Walnut Cookies

These cookies keep almost forever in a sealed container. Over time, they become softer and chewier--perfect for dunking in your tea or coffee. Makes four dozen.

INGREDIENTS
- 2 cups raw honey
- 2 cups ground walnuts
- 4 cups almond flour
- 1/2 teaspoon nutmeg
- 1/2 teaspoon ginger
- 1/2 cup dried fruit chopped

DIRECTIONS
Preheat oven to 350 degrees. Lightly grease cookie sheets, or line with parchment paper. Warm the honey in a saucepan. Let mixture cool slightly.
Sift together flour and spices. Place honey in mixing bowl; gradually add flour mixture and stir until well blended. Stir in dried chopped fruit.

Roll dough about 1/4-inch thick on a floured board; cut into squares and rectangles with a pastry wheel or sharp knife. (If you prefer, you can also make drop cookies, dropping the dough by teaspoonful.) Bake for 10 minutes.

Flourless Honey-Almond cake

INGREDIENTS Cake

- 1 1/2 cups whole almonds, toasted (see Tip)
- 4 large eggs, at room temperature (see Note), separated
- 1/2 cup honey
- 1 teaspoon vanilla extract
- 1/2 teaspoon baking soda
- 1/2 teaspoon salt

Topping

- 2 tablespoons honey
- 1/4 cup sliced almonds, toasted
- Preheat oven to 350°F. Coat a 9-inch spring form pan with cooking spray.
- Line the bottom with parchment paper and spray the paper.

DIRECTIONS

Process whole almonds in a food processor or blender until finely ground (you will have about 13/4 cups ground). Beat 4 egg yolks, 1/2 a cup honey, vanilla, baking soda and salt in a large mixing bowl with an electric mixer (or use a paddle attachment on a stand mixer) on medium speed until well combined.
Add the ground almonds and beat on low until combined.
Beat 4 egg whites in another large bowl with the electric mixer (use clean beaters on a hand-held mixer or the whisk attachment on a stand mixer) on medium speed until very foamy, white and doubled in volume, but not stiff enough to hold peaks, 1 to 2 minutes (depending on the type of mixer).
Using a rubber spatula, gently fold the egg whites into the nut mixture until just combined. Scrape the batter into the prepared pan.
Bake the cake until golden brown Use a pick or a skewer at 28 minutes, insert into the center, if it comes out clean, they are ready. Let cool in the pan for 10 minutes. Run a knife around the edge of the pan and gently remove the side ring. Let it cool completely. If desired, remove the cake from the pan bottom by gently sliding a wide spatula between the cake and the parchment paper. Carefully transfer the cake to a serving platter. To serve, drizzle the top of the cake with honey and sprinkle with sliced almonds.

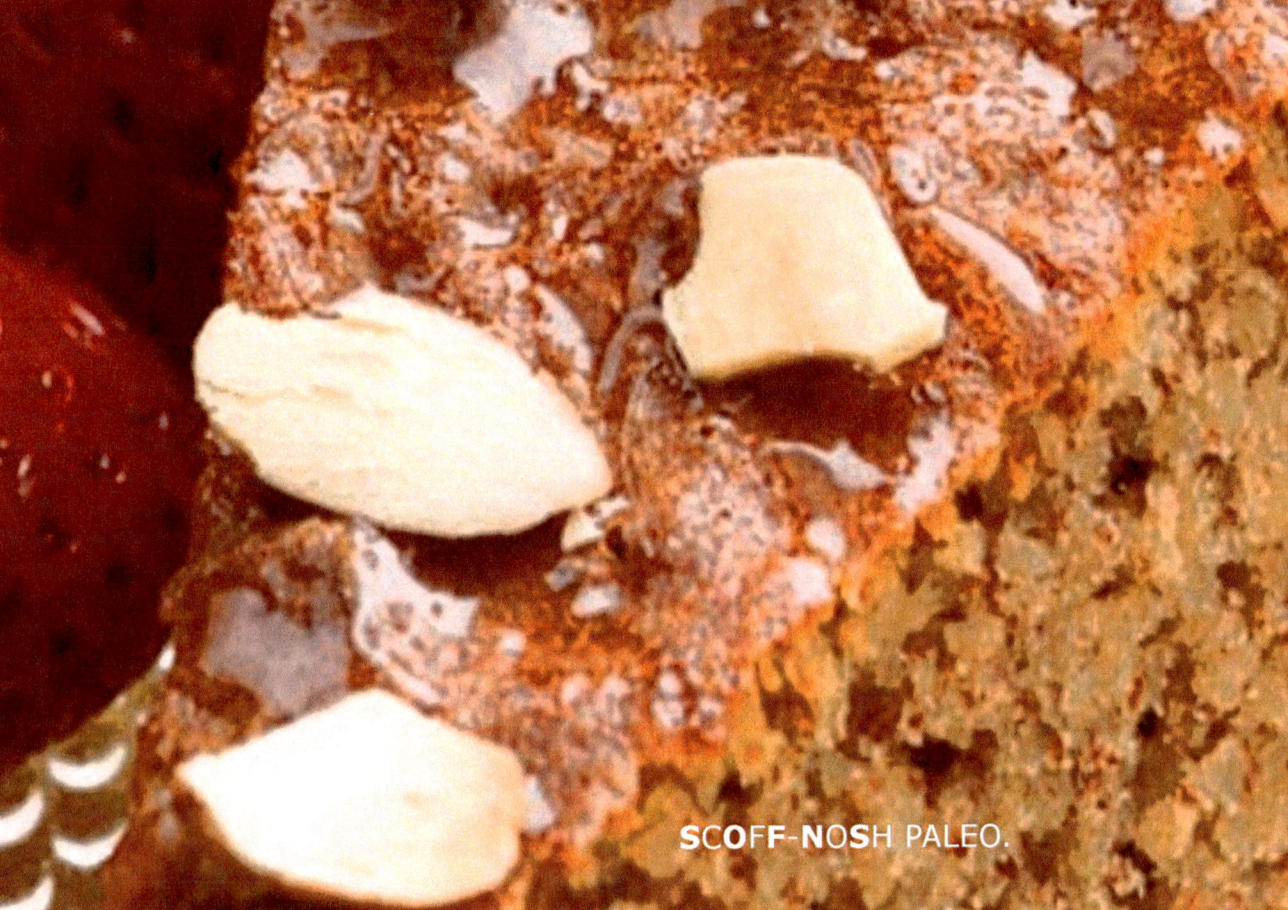

Store the cooled cake airtight at room temperature for up to 1 day. Drizzle with honey and sprinkle with almonds just before serving.
Tip: To toast whole almonds, spread on a baking sheet and bake at 350°F, Stirring once, until fragrant, 7 to 9 minutes.
To toast sliced almonds, cook in a small dry skillet over medium-low heat, stirring constantly, until fragrant and lightly browned, 2 to 4 minutes.

Note: Eggs must be at room temperature for the proteins to unwind enough to support the cake's crumb. Either set the eggs out on the counter for 15 minutes or submerge them in their shells in a bowl of lukewarm (not hot) water for 5 minutes before using.

Be careful not to overbeat the egg whites-they should be white and very foamy but not at all stiff or able to hold peaks. If you beat them too much, the cake may sink in the middle as it cools

Grain – Free Sandwich Bread

INGREDIENTS

- 1 cup of cashew butter smooth.
- 4 large eggs, separated
- 1 tablespoons honey (or 2 Tbs for sweeter dishes such as french toast)
- 21/2 teaspoons apple cider vinegar
- ¼ cup almond milk
- ¼ cup coconut Flour
- 1 Tsp. backing soda.
- ½ Tsp. sea salt

DIRECTIONS

1. Preheat oven to 300 degrees F place a small dish of water on the bottom rack.

2. Line the bottom of an 8.5×4.5 loaf pan with parchment paper, spreading a very thin coating of coconut oil on the sides of the pan.

3. Beat the cashew butter with the egg yolks, now add the honey, vinegar, and then the milk and mix.

4. Beat the egg whites in a separate bowl until peaks form using an electric hand mixer.

5. Combine all the dry ingredients into another small bowl.

6. Make sure you oven is completely preheated before adding the egg whites and the dry ingredients to the cashew butter mixture. You don't want your whites to fall, and the baking soda will activate once it hits the eggs and the vinegar.

7. Pour the dry ingredients into the wet ingredients, and then beat until they are combined. This will result in more of a wet batter mix than dough. *Make sure you get all of the sticky butter mixture off the bottom of the bowl so you don't end up with lumps.*

8. Pour the beaten egg whites into the cashew butter mixture, beating again until just combined. *Try not to over mix this part.*

9. Pour the mix into the prepared loaf pan, then IMMEDIATELY put this in the oven.

10. Bake for approximately 45-50 minutes until the top is golden brown (try the toothpick test).

Important <u>DO NOT</u> open the oven door anytime before 40 minutes, as this will allow the steam to escape and you will not get a properly risen loaf.

Remove from the oven, let cool for 20 minutes. Using a knife , free the sides from the loaf pan then flip it upside down and release onto a cooling rack. Allow bread to cool right side up for an hour before serving.

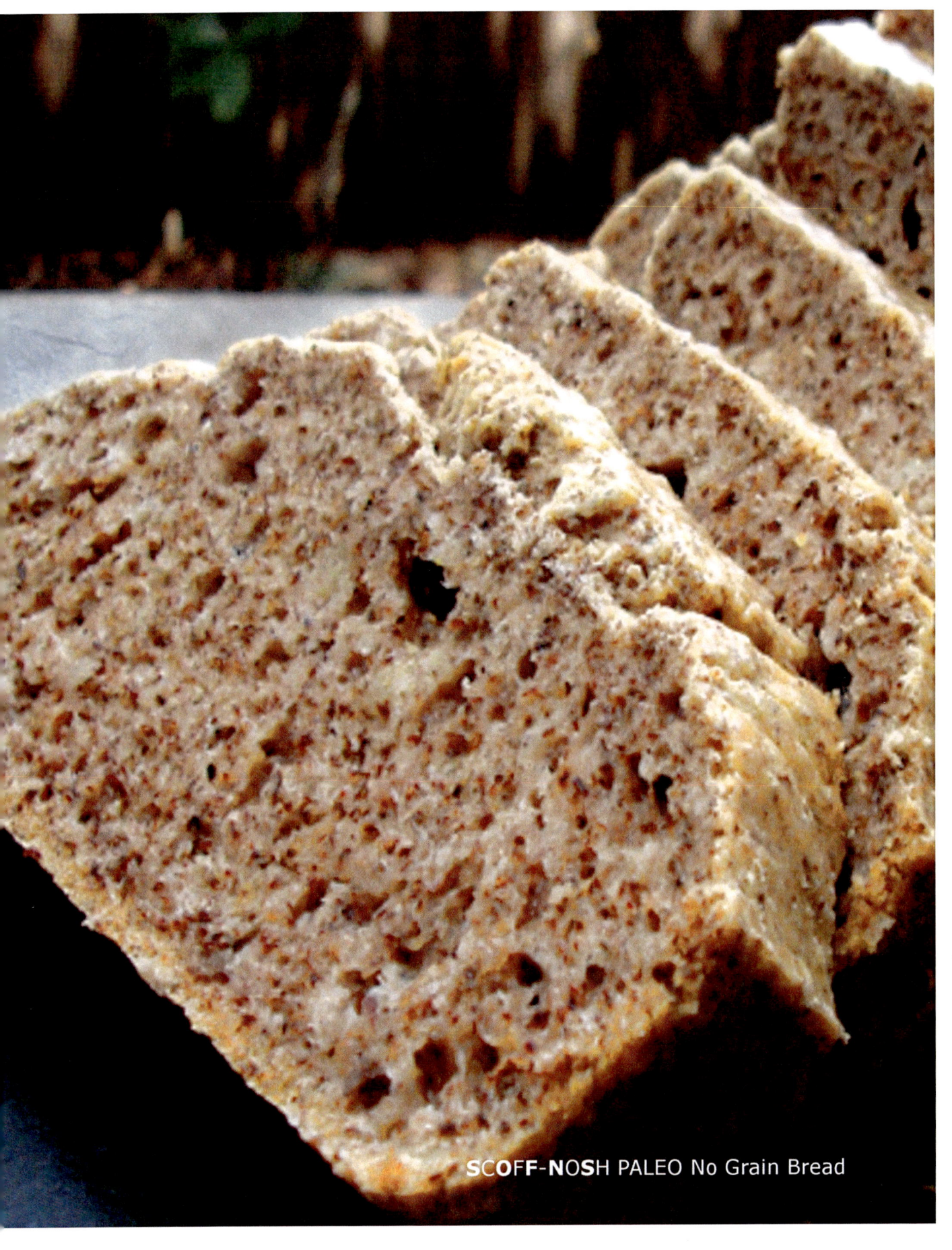

SCOFF-NOSH PALEO No Grain Bread

Walnut Cookies

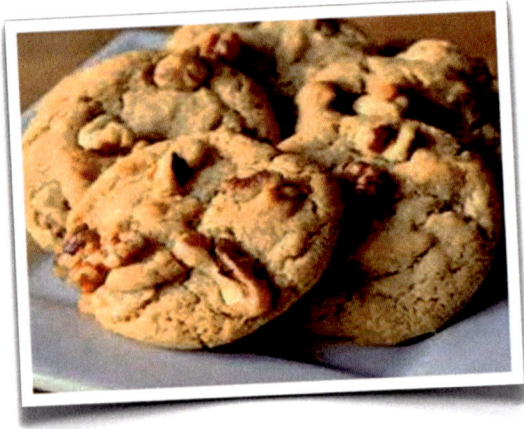

INGREDIENTS

- 2 Cups walnuts
- 1/8 cup raw, unfiltered honey (more or less to taste)
- 1 Tb. cinnamon
- 2 egg whites, whisked until frothy

DIRECTIONS

Grind the nuts and cinnamon in a blender or food processor. Now stir in the honey. Combine with the egg whites.

Now using a teaspoon place on an oiled cookie sheet.

Now Bake at 350 degrees F for 15 minutes. Cookies will be soft; do not over bake. Recipe makes about 15 cookies. This may be used as a piecrust recipe too.

CHAPTER 9

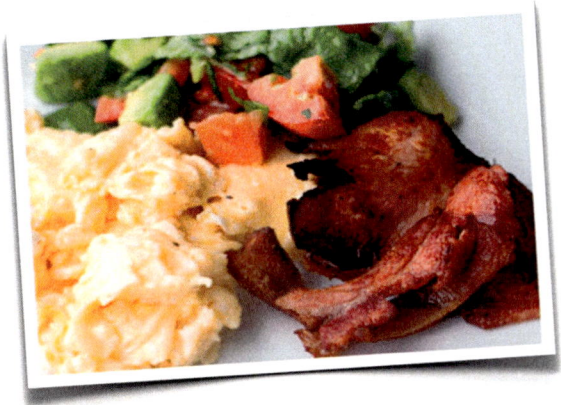

BREAKFAST PALEO RECIPES

Remember I'm sharing with your ideas mixed with some amazing recipes, but you are the *"master chef"* in your kitchen so let your creative paleo juices flow.... As you have seen the food list is extensive, so go, and be creative...

Yes I do have cheat days now and again, but, I don't feel guilty, I now eat paleo 90% of the time for sure. I don't eat dairy because I'm like 65 % of the world population, lactose intolerant. (We are the only mammal that consume the milk from any other animal) this really says to me that this is not a good option to consume in any way.

How amazing food tastes with the correct use of herbs and spices, use the herbs for some truly amazing delicious recipes for an exciting, vibrant world tour for your taste buds!!

Now any NEW food recipe we get we can convert into paleo using our new ingredients, it really is "simple dimple"... and it is a lot easier than you think.

One thing I'm sure about now ...Paleo is a sure way of having fun and enjoying delicious food without the negative health effects of processed food!

Avocado Poached Egg

With Diablo Sauce.

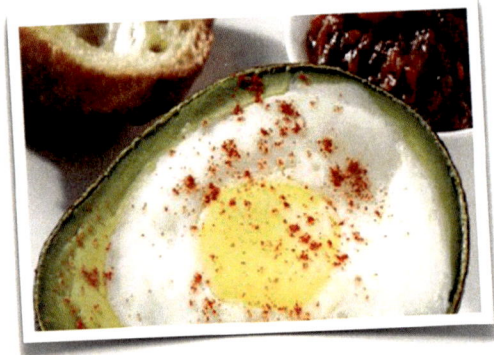

YIELD

SERVES 1 to 2 PEOPLE
TAKES 8-10 MINUTES (Diablo Sauce 20 minutes).

INGREDIENTS

- 1 Teaspoon olive oil
- 1 Garlic clove, finely chopped
- 1 (15-ounce) can fire roasted crushed tomatoes
- 1/4 Teaspoon smoked sweet paprika (plus more for garnish)
- 1/2 Teaspoon salt
- 1/4 Teaspoon pepper
- 1 Large avocado, halved and pitted
- 2 Medium eggs, room temperature chopped
- 1 (15-ounce) can, fire roasted crushed tomatoes
- 1/4 teaspoon smoked sweet paprika (plus more for garnish)
- 1/2 teaspoon salt
- 1/4 teaspoon pepper
- 1 large avocado, halved and pitted
- 2 medium eggs, room temp

DIRECTIONS

Prepare Diablo Sauce at least 20 minutes before starting eggs.

In a large skillet, heat oil until hot.

Add garlic; cook and stir until fragrant. Stir in the tomatoes, paprika, salt and pepper.

Bring to a boil; reduce to a simmer for 20 minutes, stirring frequently.

When sauce is almost finished, place a steaming basket over 1-inch of water; bring water to a simmer.

Meanwhile, cut a thin slice from the bottom of each avocado half to create a flat surface, *(so they stand steady on your plate)*.

Without breaking through the base, carefully scoop out some of the avocado flesh to create a larger indentation. Now season with salt into each avocado half, and add one egg; season with salt.

Place avocado halves in steaming basket; cover until eggs are poached, about 5 to 7 minutes.

Transfer each avocado half to a serving plate. Sprinkle with paprika, serve with the scooped avocado and Diablo Sauce.

Now sit back enjoy your Simple and healthy breakfast.

Stir-Fry Omelette

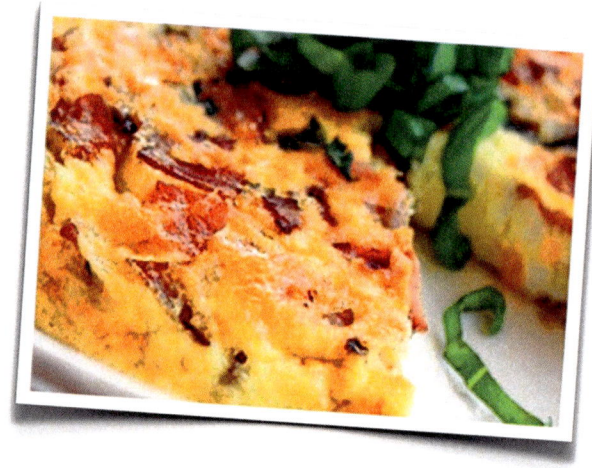

YIELD

SERVES 1 to 2 PEOPLE
TAKES 8-10 MINUTES.

INGREDIENTS

- 3 eggs, beaten
- 1 carrot, matchstick cut
- 3 scallions, diagonal sliced
- I handful tiny broccoli florets (Or other vegetables you have)
- Bits of leftover cooked chicken, pork, beef, any other meat.
- Safflower oil, Pinch of salt

DIRECTIONS

Heat oil in a wok or large cast iron skillet over medium heat, until hot enough to sizzle a drop of water. Add broccoli and carrots stir-fry 2 min. until soft.
Add cooked meat, stir fry 1 min. until heated through. Add scallions and eggs, scramble. Add salt to taste. Serve. This is wonderful for when you find yourself craving Chinese fried rice! If you should happen to have a bag of frozen peas you need to get rid of, use them in this recipe too. Add them when you add the meat.

Scrambled Eggs with Basil & Walnuts.

SERVES 1 to 2 PEOPLE
TAKES 8-10 MINUTES.

INGREDIENTS

- 3 eggs
- 1/2 cup fresh basil, chopped
- 1/3 cup walnuts, chopped.
- salt and pepper

DIRECTIONS

Whisk eggs in a bowl then place in a frying pan on medium heat, stirring constantly. When the eggs are almost cooked, add the basil and continue cooking for a further 1 minute or until eggs are fully cooked.

Add salt and pepper to taste.
Remove from heat and stir in the walnuts before serving. Whisk eggs in a bowl then place in a frying pan on medium heat, stirring
constantly.
When the eggs are almost cooked, add the basil and continue cooking for a further 1 minute or until eggs are fully cooked.
Add salt and pepper to taste.

Remove from heat and stir in the walnuts before serving. continue cooking for a further 1 minute or until eggs are fully cooked. Add salt and pepper to taste.

Remove from heat and stir in the walnuts before serving. Whisk eggs in a bowl then place in a frying pan on medium heat, stirring constantly.

When the eggs are almost cooked, add the basil and continue cooking for a further 1 minute or until eggs are fully cooked. Add salt and pepper to taste. Remove from heat and stir in the walnuts before serving.

Zucchini Pancakes

YIELD

SERVES 1 to 2 PEOPLE
TAKES 8 -10 MINUTES.

INGREDIENTS

- 1 medium stalk zucchini, ends removed and coarsely grated
- 2 eggs
- 2-3 tablespoons coconut oil
- 1 teaspoon red onion, chopped
- freshly ground black pepper
- 2-3 fresh basil leaves, minced
- 1 teaspoon coconut flour
- pinch of salt, to taste

DIRECTIONS

Grate zucchini into a bowl. Add eggs and mix thoroughly.
Start heating oil in a large skillet.

Add onion, black pepper and basil to the zucchini. If the batter looks too liquidly, add a bit of coconut flour to thicken slightly.

When the oil is hot but not smoking, put a forkful of batter into the pan, immediately mashing it down with a fork to spread the batter and form thin pancakes that can crisp easily. Repeat until pan is full. Don't worry if the pancakes run together.
When the pancakes are golden brown or deeper brown on the underside, flip them over and cook on the second side. If they have stuck together, cut them in the skillet and flip them individually. When golden brown on the second side, remove pancakes. Drain on paper towels.

Blueberry and Walnut Pancakes

YIELD

SERVES 1

TAKES 8-10 MINUTES.

INGREDIENTS

- 1/2 cup walnut meal (finely ground walnuts, should look like a course flour)
- A little sea salt
- ½ teaspoon baking powder
- 1 whole organic egg
- 1/2 cup pure water
- 1 1/2 teaspoons walnut oil
- Chopped walnuts
- Blueberries

DIRECTIONS

Cook each pancake in a little walnut oil, flip once and serve with a very small amount of warm, pure maple syrup.

....

Apple, streusel Muffins

YIELD

SERVES 3-6

TAKES 45 MINUTES.

INGREDIENTS

- 3 large green apples granny smiths work best. (chop these into ½ inch random pieces, 2 cups)
- 3 tablespoons of warm water
- 2 teaspoons of cinnamon
- 6-9 eggs
- 11/2 tablespoons butter or use coconut oil, melted.
- 3 tablespoons of coconut milk

- 11/2 tablespoons of coconut flour
- ¼ teaspoon of baking soda
- 1 pinch of sea salt

This amazing recipe is so versatile and can be re-created into so many different recipes. Substitute the apple for bananas, or pears. Add a small cup of chopped nuts for amazing texture and a serving of healthy fats.

DIRECTIONS

Preheat oven to 350 F

Using a medium sized skillet, sauté the apples, add the water and 11/2 teaspoons of cinnamon until the apples are like chunky applesauce / apple pie filling. I like mine chunky to do this to suit your consistency.

Once done allow the mixture to cool down.

Take a medium sized mixing bowl, whisk the eggs, butter, coconut milk, coconut flour, ½ teaspoon of cinnamon, baking soda and a pinch of salt until all the ingredients are wall well combined. Now add the cooled apples saving a ¼ cup to garnish. Combine the ingredients then spoon the mixture into lined muffin tins, about ¼ cup. Then gently add the garnish on top of the mix, about a teaspoon per muffin. Place in the oven for 40 minutes. You can use the tooth pick test to make sure there are fully cooked through the middle. Enjoy... by far one of my favorite recipes.

···

Fluffy Coconut Flour Pancakes

YIELD

SERVES 2-3

TAKES 6-8 MINUTES.

INGREDIENTS

You can also add other ingredients like cinnamon or fruit as desired. Keep the pancakes small and watch them so they don't burn.

- 4 eggs, room temp
- 1 cup coconut milk
- 2 teaspoons vanilla extract

- 1 tablespoon honey or a pinch of stevia [will be dry with stevia]
- 1/2 cup coconut flour
- 1 teaspoon baking soda
- 1/4 teaspoon sea salt
- Coconut oil for frying

DIRECTIONS

Preheat griddle over medium-low heat. In a small bowl beat eggs until frothy, about two minutes. Mix in milk, vanilla, and honey or stevia.

In a medium-sized bowl combine coconut flour, baking soda, and sea salt and whisk together. Stir wet mixture into dry until coconut flour is mixed.
Grease pan with butter or coconut oil. Ladle a few tablespoons of batter into pan for each pancake. Spread out slightly with the back of a spoon.
The pancakes should be 2-3 inches in diameter and thick. Cook for a few minutes on each side, until the tops dry out slightly and the bottoms start to brown. Flip and cook an additional 2-3 minutes.
Serve hot with coconut oil, honey, syrup, or fruit.

Additional Info:

- Add chopped nuts.
- Substituted baking powder for the baking soda (aluminum free).
- I used 1/2 tsp. of baking soda and 1/2 tsp. baking powder.
I used Baking Powder as well but you need 3 teaspoons not 1 and you can also, reduce the salt when you use Baking Powder.
The key for those who are struggling with thin pancakes is to let it sit for 5 min. Coconut flour has to absorb the liquid and does so slowly.

Nut Flour Muffins

YIELD

SERVES 3-4
TAKES 18 MINUTES.

INGREDIENTS

- 1 1/4 cups of nut flour: walnuts, almonds, sunflower seeds, etc.

- 2 eggs
- 1 banana
- 1/8 cup of coconut oil
- handful of berries or fruit: blueberries, apple grated, peach...

DIRECTIONS

Put everything except fruit in a food processor and add fruit before pouring into greased muffin tins. Bake @ 350 about 12-15 min.

Almond Muffins

YIELD

SERVES 3-4
TAKES 22 MINUTES.

INGREDIENTS

- 1 cup almond butter
- 1 cup sliced raw almonds
- 1 cup pure coconut milk
- 2 cups unsweetened shredded coconut
- 3 eggs

DIRECTIONS

Beat all the ingredients together in a large mixing bowl and pour in muffin cups. Cook at 400 F for 15 minutes.

Doughnut & Banana

YIELD

SERVES 2-4
TAKES 14 MINUTES.

INGREDIENTS

About 2-3 cups almond flour
2 eggs
1 banana
1/8 cup of coconut oil

DIRECTIONS

Mix all ingredients, using just 1 cup almond flour, in a food processor.
Place in a bowl and continue adding almond flour, stirring frequently, until the dough has reached a consistency that you can shape it into 1-1/4 inch balls. Deep fry in coconut oil until golden brown. Watch them, they burn quickly. Roll in topping (honey, chopped nuts, cinnamon, toasted coconut) and eat as soon as cool enough, or the next day (somehow they are not as good in that in-between time). Enjoy with spiced cider.

Chicken Coconut Nuggets

YIELD

SERVES 2-3
TAKES 15 MINUTES.

INGREDIENTS

- 2 lb. chicken, boneless and skinless - breasts or thighs
- 1/3 cup coconut flour
- 4 eggs
- 1 1/3 cups shred coconut
- 1/2 teaspoon garlic powder
- 1/4 teaspoon onion powder
- 1/2 teaspoon paprika
- 1/4 teaspoon black pepper
- 1 teaspoon salt
- 1/2 cup coconut oil - divided

DIRECTIONS

Cut thawed chicken into desired length strips, pat dry with paper towel.

Place coconut flour in a flat dish wide enough for dipping.
Put eggs in another flat dish and whisk.

Put the rest of the dry ingredients in a third flat dish; stir ingredients
until mixed.
Line up dipping bowls and dip chicken strips first in flour, then in egg, then in
coating mixture.
Heat 1/4 cup coconut oil in a frying pan. Fry strips on medium heat until done,
about 4-5 minutes on each side, adding oil as needed.

....

Paleo Breakfast Sausage Patties

YIELD
SERVES 2-3
TAKES 15 MINUTES.

INGREDIENTS

- 1 Beaten Egg
- 1/3 Cup Finely Chopped Onion
- 1/4 Cup finely snipped dried or 1/2 cup fresh chopped apples (Optional)
- 2 Tbs. Parsley flakes or snipped fresh parsley
- 1/2 tsp. sea salt
- 1/2 tsp. ground sage
- 1/4 tsp. ground nutmeg
- 1/4 tsp. black pepper
- 1/8 tsp. red cayenne pepper (this is for mild sausage, add more if you like it hot)
- 1/2 lb. ground pork (can also substitute ground beef, turkey, or chicken)

DIRECTIONS

Combine all ingredients in large bowl and mix well. Form into patties and
grill or pan fry. Enjoy delicious tasting sausage

Breakfast or Country Sausage

YIELD

SERVES Many
TAKES 20 MINUTES.

INGREDIENTS

- 10 lbs. pork shoulder
- 4 Tb. salt
- 1 1/2 Tb. white pepper
- 2 1/2 Tb. sage
- 1 Tb. nutmeg
- 1 Tb. thyme
- 1 1/2 tsp. ginger
- 1/2 Tb. cayenne pepper
- 2 Cups ice water

DIRECTIONS

Trim the fat off the pork shoulder, if you like lean sausage, or leave it
on if you like more flavor. Always make certain that your meat is free of bone and
glands. Use the 1/8" grinding plate, grinding the meat only once.
To the ground meat, mix in the dry spices first. Then add the ice water. Mix
thoroughly. Bulk sausage is easily made into patties, or you can use 22-24mm
lamb casings for the challenge of making link sausage. Wrap the finished product
in freezer paper for long-term storage.

....

Avocado Fruit Salad with Lemonade Dressing

YIELD

SERVES 2-4
TAKES 20 MINUTES.

INGREDIENTS

- 1/4 cup fresh lemon juice
- 4 teaspoons honey
- 1/4 teaspoon ground chili piquin (optional)
- 3/4 cup fresh pineapple cubes (about 3/4-inch)
- 3/4 cup fresh papaya cubes (about 3/4-inch)
- 3/4 cup fresh quartered strawberries
- 3/4 cup jicama cubes (about 1/2-inch)
- 1 medium jalapeño, seeded and finely chopped
- 2 tablespoons coarsely chopped mint
- 1 firm-ripe avocado, halved, pitted, peeled and cut into 3/4-inch chunks

DIRECTIONS

In a medium bowl, whisk together the lemon juice, honey and chili piquin, if using. Stir in the pineapple, papaya, strawberries, jicama, jalapeño and mint until evenly coated with the lemonade dressing. Gently fold in the avocado and serve.

Fresh Spinach Salad 1 lb. fresh spinach, washed, drained and torn into desired pieces 1 can sliced water chestnuts 1 lb. fresh mushrooms, sliced thinly 1/2 lb. bacon, cooked and crumbled
4 hardboiled eggs, sliced.
Make sure spinach has been well drained and isn't watery.
Combine all above salad ingredients in a large bowl. Chill.

· ·

Coconut Flour Bread

YIELD

SERVES 2-4
TAKES 44 MINUTES.

INGREDIENTS

- 6 eggs
- 1/2 cup melted coconut oil
- 1-2 tablespoons honey (optional, I usually leave it out)

- 1/2 teaspoon sea salt
- 3/4 cup coconut flour

DIRECTIONS

Mix all ingredients together and pour into a small oiled loaf pan. Bake at 350 degrees F for 40 minutes.

Turn the loaf out and cool completely on a rack before serving.

....

Coconut Flour Flax Bread

YIELD

SERVES 2-4
TAKES 46 MINUTES.

INGREDIENTS

- 1/2 cup coconut flour, sifted
- 1/2 cup flax seeds, ground [or chia seeds, unground]
- 1/2 teaspoon salt [or less]
- 1 teaspoon baking soda
- 5 eggs
- 1/4 cup coconut oil, melted
- 1/8 cup water (or coconut milk for a moister bread)
- 1 teaspoon apple cider vinegar [or coconut water vinegar or lemon juice]

DIRECTIONS

Preheat oven to 325F. Grease a small loaf pan (7 3/4" × 4 1/2" × 3" H).
Mix all the dry ingredients together.
Combine all the wet ingredients.
Add the dry ingredients to the wet and beat well. Batter will be thick.
Pour into loaf pan and bake for 40 minutes or until toothpick comes out Clean.
Cool completely before slicing.

Pumpkin Bread.

INGREDIENTS

- 1 cup almond flour*
- 1/4 cup coconut flour
- 1/2 teaspoon baking powder
- 1/2 teaspoon salt
- 3 tablespoons pumpkin pie spice
- 1/2 teaspoon high-quality cinnamon
- 4 large eggs
- 1/2 cup coconut oil, melted
- 1/2 cup pumpkin puree
- 2 tablespoons maple syrup/honey.
- 10-15 drops vanilla stevia [optional]
- 1/8 cup pumpkin seeds

DIRECTIONS

Preheat oven to 350 F.

In a medium bowl, mix the almond and coconut flours together, along with the baking powder, salt, pumpkin pie spice, and cinnamon. Set the dry mixture aside. In a mixer bowl, cream the eggs and the coconut oil together until smooth, then add the pumpkin, maple syrup, and stevia. Mix the wet ingredients until thoroughly combined.

Slowly add the dry ingredients. Mix until fully combined.

Oil a small loaf pan with coconut oil and then our batter into pan.

Sprinkle the pumpkin seeds on top. Bake at 350 for 35-50 minutes. Check the loaf with a toothpick at 30 minutes. If it doesn't come out clean, continue baking. Remove from oven and let cool for about an hour before removing from the pan. Let the loaf cool completely before cutting. Use a lightly serrated knife to cut.

Additionally. You can grind your own almond flour by placing whole peeled almonds in a blender/food processor and blend until a consistency is reached.

Coconut Cinnamon Banana Bread

YIELD

SERVES 4-6
TAKES up to 38 MINUTES.

INGREDIENTS

- 8 eggs
- 2 mashed ripe bananas
- 2 teaspoons vanilla
- 5 teaspoons cinnamon
- 1/2 teaspoon salt
- 1/2 cup melted coconut oil
- 5 tablespoons maple syrup or honey
- 1/2 cup shredded coconut
- 3/4 cup coconut flour

DIRECTIONS

Preheat your oven to 350 degrees F.

Mix all ingredients well together until fully combined.

Pour into 6 mini loaf pans, 12 muffin tins, or small loaf tin Bake for 25-35 minutes (muffins take less time than mini loaves) or until it tests done.

Porridge Without Grain.

YIELD

SERVES 1

PREP TIME 3 MINUTES | **TOTAL TIME** 6 MINUTES

INGREDIENTS

- 1 Handful Fresh berries / strawberries or chopped banana.
- ¼ cup of shredded coconut (unsweetened)
- 2 tablespoons of almond butter
- 6-8 Tablespoons of coconut milk (try Full fat)
- ¼ teaspoon of Vanilla extract
- ½ teaspoon of cinnamon spice
- 1 teaspoon of organic honey or maple syrup.

DIRECTIONS

Mix all the ingredients into a small mixing bowl. Then transfer ingredients into a saucepan on low and heat until warm.
Serve and add fruit garnish to your taste.

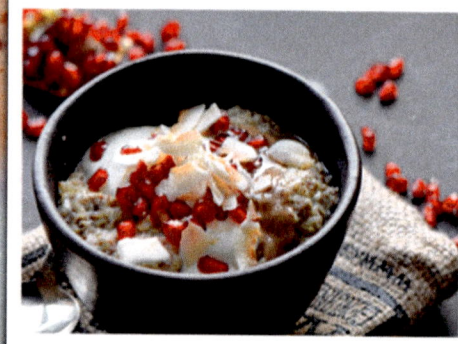

SCOFF-NOSH PALEO No Grain Porridge

CHAPTER 10

PALEO BEVERAGE RECIPES

My selection of amazing quick and easy to make paleo drinks. Try to experiment with them too!

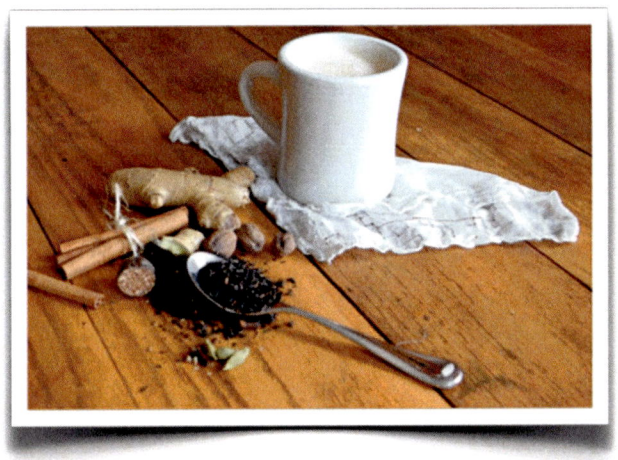

Chai – tea

YIELD

SERVES 6-8

PREP TIME 4 MINUTES | **TOTAL TIME** 8 MINUTES

INGREDIENTS

In a sauce pan with a tight fitting lid combine the following:

- 8 cups water
- 6-10 quarter sized slices of fresh ginger root
- 10-15 cardamom pods, cracked open
- 1 teaspoon of fennel seeds
- 4 cloves
- 1-2 pieces of dried orange rind
- 8-10 black peppercorns

DIRECTIONS

Bring to a boil. Reduce heat and simmer, covered for at least 20 minutes. Simmer longer for a richer, spicier flavor. This tea can be sweetened with raw honey. You can also add almond milk or coconut milk or add one green tea bag for a stronger tea.

....

Cranberry Tea

YIELD

SERVES 4-6

PREP TIME 4 MINUTES | **TOTAL TIME** 6 MINUTES

INGREDIENTS

- 1 lb. cranberries
- 1/2 cup honey
- 2-1/2 qt. water
- 4 cinnamon sticks
- 2 tsp. whole cloves
- 1 cup orange juice

DIRECTIONS

In covered saucepan, combine cranberries, honey, and water; simmer until cranberries pop; add cinnamon sticks and cloves; continue to simmer until it smells good. Add orange juice. Strain and keep juice (use pulp in other recipes). 1 Tbs. lemon juice can be added to tea, if desired. Serve warm not hot.

Russian Tea

INGREDIENTS

- 1 Cup of green tea
- 1/4 Cup fresh squeezed orange juice
- 1 to 2 teaspoons spiced honey to taste.

DIRECTIONS

In saucepan, combine ingredients and simmer until it smells good.

....

Alternative Beverage "Coffee Substitute"

YIELD

SERVES 4-6
PREP TIME 10 MINUTES | **TOTAL TIME** 12 MINUTES

INGREDIENTS

- 2 cups water
- 1 Tbs roasted chicory root
- 1 Tbs dried dandelion root (not roasted)
- 1/2 tsp cardamon seed (should be out of the husk, but not ground)

DIRECTIONS

Put water in a pan. Add roasted chicory root, dandelion root, and cardamom seed. Simmer gently 10 minutes. Strain and enjoy. I have found this is pleasant to drink. Does it taste exactly like coffee? No, but it is dark and tasty.

Warming Winter Spice Tea

YIELD

SERVES 4-6

PREP TIME 4 MINUTES | **TOTAL TIME** 8 MINUTES

INGREDIENTS

- 2 parts roasted dandelion root
- 1/2 part cinnamon bark
- 1/2 part dried gingerroot
- 1/2 part decorticated (hulled) cardamom seeds
- 1/2 part star anise
- Raw honey to taste

DIRECTIONS

Slowly heat 4 cups of spring water in a pot. Put the ingredients into a mortar and pestle then crush the herbs slightly. Or you can put them in a blender and turn it on briefly, just enough to cut and release some of the aromas.

....

Mulled Cider

YIELD

SERVES 4-6

PREP TIME 8 MINUTES | **TOTAL TIME** 42 MINUTES

INGREDIENTS

- 2 quarts apple cider or juice
- 1 orange, sliced
- 1 lemon, sliced
- 2 Tablespoon maple syrup or raw honey
- 4 sticks cinnamon
- 6 whole cloves
- 1/4 teaspoon of nutmeg
- 1/4 teaspoon powdered ginger.

DIRECTIONS

In large saucepan, combine all of the ingredients. Bring mixture to a boil. Reduce the heat to low, and simmer the cider for 30-40 minutes. Strain and serve hot.

....

Home-Made Strawberry Lemonade

YIELD

SERVES 6-8

PREP TIME 10 MINUTES | **TOTAL TIME** (see directions)

INGREDIENTS

- 8 cups water
- 1 cup of fresh-cut strawberries
- 1 cup frozen strawberries
- honey to your taste
- 1 cup lemon juice
- 2 lemons sliced

DIRECTIONS

In a large container, combine 4 cups of water and the fresh and frozen strawberries. Let them soak in the sun for 3-4 hours
In a separate container, combine the lemon juice, sliced lemons and water. Chill for 3-4 hours to allow the lemon juice soak through. Mix the 2 containers together, and add honey to your taste. Serve over crushed ice.

....

Apple Lemonade

YIELD

SERVES 2

PREP TIME 2 MINUTES | **TOTAL TIME** 4 MINUTES

INGREDIENTS

- 2 cups unsweetened apple juice
- 4 tablespoons pure lemon juice

DIRECTIONS

Combine both juices. Chill. Serve over crushed ice.

....

Tomato Sauce / Juice

YIELD

SERVES 1-2

PREP TIME 3 MINUTES | **TOTAL TIME** 5 MINUTES

INGREDIENTS

- Whole ripe organic tomatoes
- Lemon Juice
- Pinch Salt

DIRECTIONS

Since many classic recipes call for tomato juice or tomato sauce, it's necessary to know with you can make your own rather than rely on the canned varieties that contain additives. To make tomato juice, simply puree tomatoes in a blender, add lemon juice and salt. Strain the mixture for juice and retain the pulp and a little juice to use in recipes calling for tomato juice. ☺

CHAPTER 11

POULTRY RECIPES FOR PALEO

Sage and Garlic Roasted Chicken

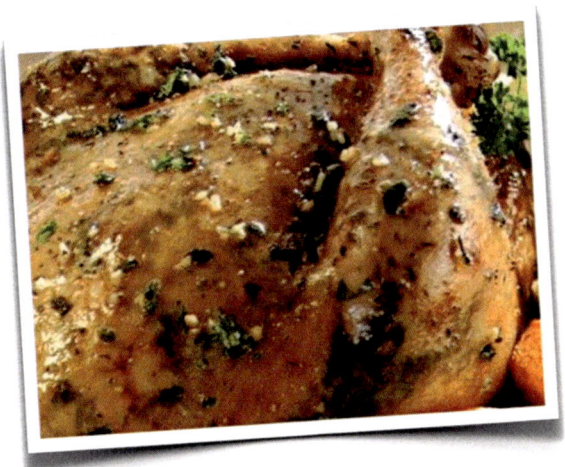

YIELD

SERVES 3-4

PREP TIME Varies | **TOTAL TIME** Varies

INGREDIENTS

- 1 4-5 lb. young chicken
- 1 Tablespoon. dried sage
- 4-5 cloves garlic, peeled and halved length-wise
- 1 Tbs. olive oil / salt and pepper

DIRECTIONS

Preheat oven to 375. Wash chicken inside and out, pat dry with paper towels.
In a small bowl, whisk together sage, oil, salt and pepper. Rub this mixture under the skin of the breast and on the skin all over the chicken. Insert garlic slices under the skin of the breast, drum and thigh. Place chicken, breast side down, on lightly greased pan. Roast for 30 minutes, then turn the chicken breast side up and continue roasting until internal temperature reaches 180.*

North African Roast Chicken Thighs (With Raisins, Almonds, and Apricots)

In this dish we see a commonly used technique for cooking with spices, which is to add them at the sauté stage and sweat them to bring out their flavors.

YIELD

SERVES 4-6 as an Entre'
PREP TIME 15 MINUTES | **TOTAL TIME** 55 MINUTES

INGREDIENTS

- 12 skinless chicken thighs (bones in)
- Salt and freshly cracked black pepper to taste
- 2 tablespoons virgin olive oil
- 1 yellow onion, thinly sliced
- 1 tablespoon minced garlic
- 2 small to medium-sized sweet potatoes, peeled and cut into bite-size chunks
- 1 tablespoon minced ginger
- 1 tablespoon ground cumin
- 1 tablespoon ground cinnamon
- 1 tablespoon ground coriander
- 1 teaspoon ground turmeric
- 1 teaspoon paprika
- 2 teaspoons salt
- 4 cups chicken stock
- 2 tablespoons lemon juice (about 1/2 lemon)
- 1/4 cup raisins
- 1/4 cup dried apricots, chopped
- 1/4 cup blanched almonds, roughly chopped
- 1 tablespoon minced fresh red or green chili pepper.

DIRECTIONS

Heat the oven to 350°F. Sprinkle the chicken thighs with salt and pepper.
In a large sauté pan, heat the olive oil over medium heat until hot but not smoking, add the chicken thighs and cook, moving around every couple of minutes, until well browned on all sides, 5 to 7 minutes. Remove and set aside.

Add the onion slices to the sauté pan and sauté over medium heat, stirring frequently, until they begin to brown, 5 to 7 minutes. Add the garlic and cook, stirring frequently, 1 additional minute.

Add the sweet potatoes, ginger, spices, and salt and cook, still stirring frequently, for 1 more
minute. Add the stock, reserved chicken thighs, and all the remaining ingredients and bring to a boil.
Cover the sauté pan, put it in the preheated oven, and cook until the chicken thighs are tender and cooked through, 20 to 25 minutes. Season with salt and pepper and serve.

....

Lebanese Chicken

YIELD

SERVES 6-8
PREP TIME 15 MINUTES | **TOTAL TIME** 60 MINUTES

INGREDIENTS

- 3/4 c Lemon juice
- 8 lg Garlic clove(s), minced
- 2 Tbs Thyme, minced or
- 2 tsp. Dried thyme
- 1 Tbs Paprika
- 1 1/2 tsp. Ground cumin
- 3/4 tsp. Cayenne pepper
- 2 Chickens (3 lb. each) Split lengthwise, backbones

Removed and discarded Lemon wedges to garnish.

DIRECTIONS

Whisk lemon juice, minced garlic, thyme, paprika, cumin, and cayenne pepper in a small bowl. Place the chicken in 13 x 9 x 2-inch glass baking dish. Pour the marinade over; turn chicken to coat. Cover and refrigerate at least 6 hours or overnight, turning occasionally.

Preheat oven to 425 F. Transfer chicken and marinade to large roasting pan. Season chicken with salt and pepper. Bake until chicken is golden brown and cooked through, basting occasionally with pan juices, about 50 min.

Transfer chicken to plates. Garnish with lemon wedges. Pass pan juices separately.

Baked Greek Chicken

YIELD

SERVES 6-8
PREP TIME 15 MINUTES | **TOTAL TIME** 50 MINUTES

YIELD

SERVES 6-8
TAKES 50 MINUTES

INGREDIENTS

- 1 whole broiler/fryer chicken, about 5 lbs., cut in 6
- 3/4 tsp. salt
- 2 lemons
- 3 cloves garlic, minced
- 1 Tbs fresh oregano, chopped
- 1/8 tsp. black pepper
- 1 Tbs olive oil
- 1 fennel bulb (about 1-1/2 lbs.) trimmed, cored and sliced
- 1/3 c pitted kalamata olives, halved

DIRECTIONS

Pre-heat oven to 425 degrees F. Pat chicken dry. Loosen skin and sprinkle 1/4 tsp. salt underneath the skin. Grate the zest of 1 lemon, cut lemon in heal and juice. In small bowl, stir together 2 tsp. of the zest, 2 Tablespoons of the lemon juice, remaining 1/2 tsp. salt, the garlic, oregano and pepper.

Tuck half of this mixture under skin of chicken.
Cut peel off second lemon; chop fruit into pieces.

Add olive oil to remaining herb mixture in the bowl. Toss with sliced fennel and chopped lemon. Transfer to a large baking dish. Top with chicken pieces and bake at 425 for 40 minutes, or until meat registers 160 degrees.
Remove from the oven. Sprinkle the olives on top.

....

Chicken Thighs with Flax Seed Coating

YIELD

SERVES 3-4

PREP TIME 20 MINUTES | **TOTAL TIME** 55 MINUTES

INGREDIENTS

- I whole medium chicken or 6 Chicken thighs,
- ½ cup flax seed,
- 4 crushed garlic cloves
- 1 1/2 tablespoons of salt (to taste)
- 1 Tablespoon of pepper (to taste),
- 4-6 sprigs of sage or Rosemary

DIRECTIONS

A simple recipe to coat a chicken or chicken thighs with ground up flax seeds and bake chicken as normal.
You can make a coating of ground flax seed, garlic, salt, pepper, and dried herbs sage or rosemary. You can alter the herbs to your liking. You can dip in egg first to get the coating to stick better. Bake at
350° for 20 min. turn over and cook another 20 minutes.

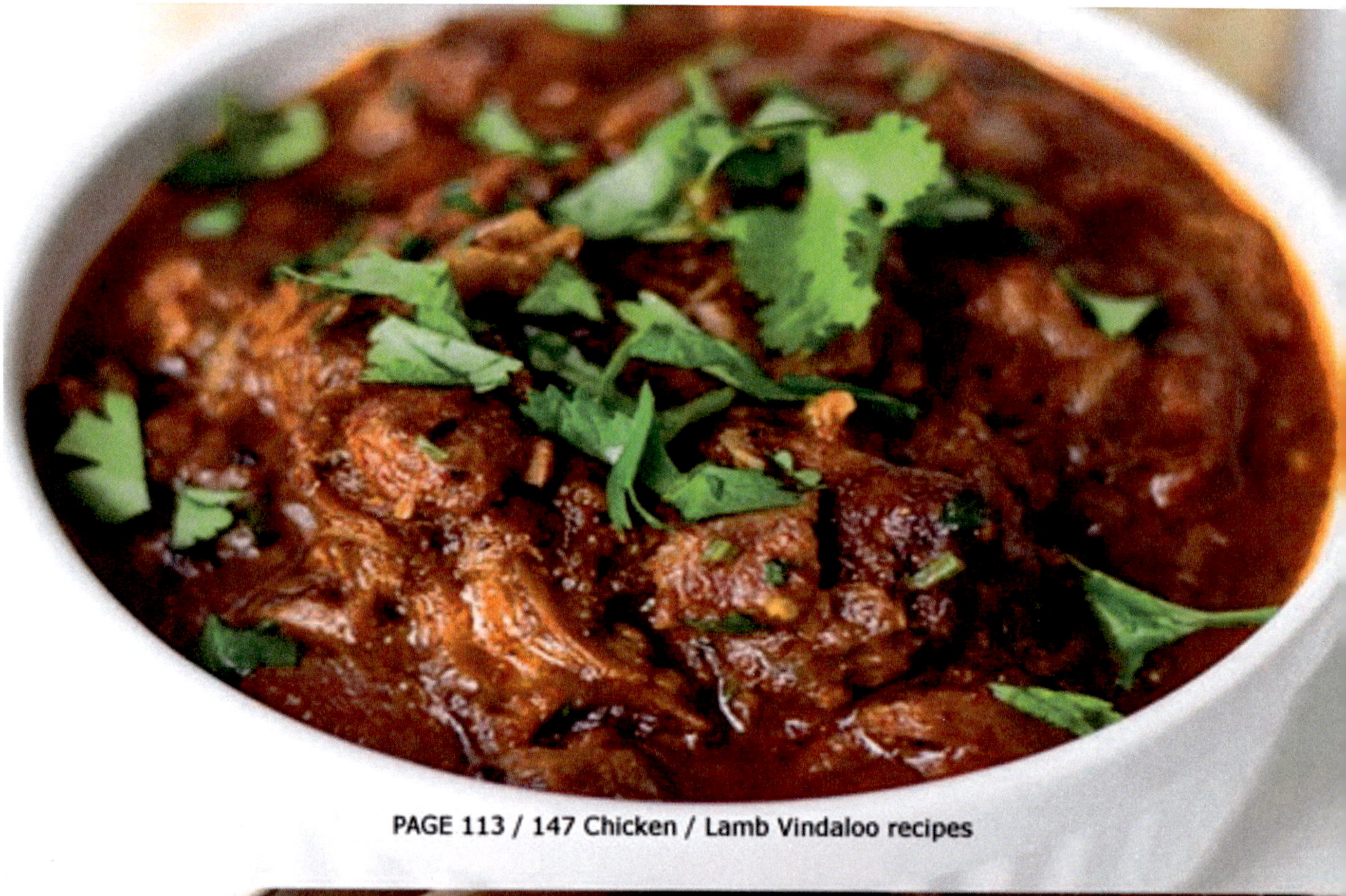

PAGE 113 / 147 Chicken / Lamb Vindaloo recipes

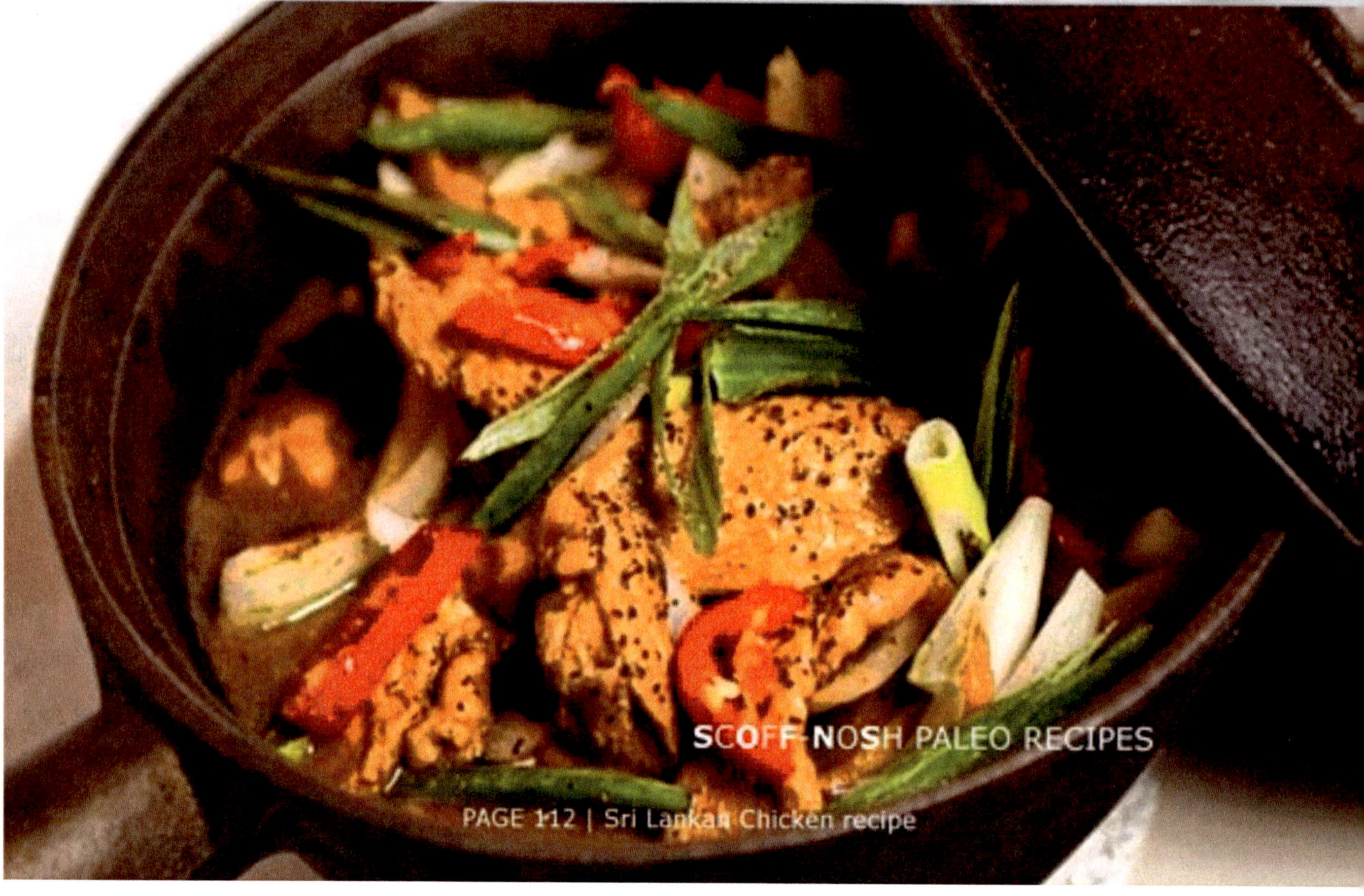

SCOFF-NOSH PALEO RECIPES

PAGE 112 | Sri Lankan Chicken recipe

SLOW COOKER RECIPES

Whole Chicken in a Crock Pot

The most delicious whole chicken recipe I have tasted. To slow cook a whole chicken until it is falling-off-the bone.

YIELD
SERVES 4

PREP TIME 12 MINUTES | **TOTAL TIME** 4-5 HOURS*

INGREDIENTS

- 2 teaspoons paprika
- 1 teaspoon salt
- 1 teaspoon onion powder
- 1 teaspoon thyme –or–
- 3-4 long sprigs fresh rosemary
- 1/2 teaspoon garlic powder
- 1/4 teaspoon cayenne (red) pepper
- 1/4 teaspoon black pepper
- 1 Medium size onion
- 1 large chicken

DIRECTIONS

Combine the dried spices in a small bowl.

Loosely chop the onion and place it in the bottom of the slow cooker.

Remove any giblets from the chicken and then rub the spice mixture all over. You can even put some of the spices inside the cavity and under the skin covering the breasts.

Put prepared chicken on top of the onions in the slow cooker, cover it, and turn it on to high. There is no need to add any liquid.

Cook for 4 - 5 hours (for a 3-4 pound chicken) or until the chicken is falling off the bone.

Sri Lankan Chicken Slow cooker

YIELD
SERVES 4
PREP TIME 10 MINUTES | **TOTAL TIME** 4-6 HOURS

INGREDIENTS

- 4-5 chicken breasts
- 1 medium white onion, diced
- 1" cube fresh ginger root, crushed (about 2 tablespoons)
- 4 Thai Chili's (Try two jalapenos and two Serrano's) - thinly sliced
- 4 cloves garlic
- 1 Tablespoon coriander
- 1 teaspoon turmeric
- Cayenne - a pinch if you like it mild up to 1/2 Tbs. to get it zinging. Also consider Paprika and /or Chili Powder
- 1 Tbs. curry powder or 1/4 cup fresh curry leaves (1 pandan leaf)
- 1 can coconut milk
- 2 teaspoon coconut oil
- 2 tablespoon lemon juice.
- 2-3 Tablespoon of White Vinegar. Season and pulls all the flavours together.

DIRECTIONS

Using a large skillet over medium - high heat and the sauté your onions, peppers, and garlic in 2tsp of coconut oil until the onion starts to become clear. Now add ALL your spices and keep cooking until it becomes very aromatic and gets a toasted smell. This will greatly enhance the flavor and strength of the spices.
Take the vegetable and spice mixture and pour into your slow cooker.
Pour in one can of coconut milk and your lemon juice. Now mix well. Place your chicken breasts in the mixture and ladle the sauce over the tops. Cook on low in your slow cooker for 6 hours or on high for 4 hours.

Crockpot Italian Chicken

YIELD

SERVES 4

PREP TIME 10 MINUTES | **TOTAL TIME** 4-6 HOURS

INGREDIENTS

- 12 boneless, skinless chicken thighs, cut into 1-inch pieces
- 2 14.5 oz. cans tomatoes with Italian herbs
- 2 cups cubed zucchini
- 1 cup pearl onions, peeled
- 1 cup baby carrots
- 2 tablespoons tomato paste
- 4 cloves garlic, chopped
- 1 teaspoon raw honey
- 1 teaspoon red pepper flakes

DIRECTIONS

Combine all ingredients in crockpot. Stir to mix.
Cook on low setting 6 to 10 hours or until done.

Crock Pot Chicken Vindaloo

YIELD

SERVES 4

PREP TIME 10 MINUTES | **TOTAL TIME** 4-6 HOURS

INGREDIENTS

- 3 tablespoons lemon or lime juice
- 3 garlic cloves, minced
- 1 1/2 tablespoons fresh ginger
- 3/4 tablespoon curry powder
- 1 tablespoon ground cumin
- 1/4 teaspoon ground cardamom

- 1/4 teaspoon ground cloves
- 1/4 teaspoon ground hot pepper
- 1 tablespoon mustard seeds
- 2 tablespoons olive oil
- 1 cup tomato sauce
- 1 cinnamon stick
- 1 small onion, chopped
- 3 boneless skinless chicken breast halves, quartered
- 2 tablespoons fresh parsley, chopped

DIRECTIONS

Puree first 10 ingredients in a blender.

Pour into the crock pot, add tomato sauce, cinnamon stick, onion and mix well.

Add chicken and turn to cover.

Cook on low for 5 hours.

Sprinkle with chopped parsley before serving.

....

Crockpot ENGLISH STYLE Chicken

YIELD

SERVES 4

PREP TIME 10 MINUTES | **TOTAL TIME** 4-6 HOURS

INGREDIENTS

- 1 Medium sized organic chicken
- 2 tablespoons of butter.
- 1 1/2 tablespoons rosemary fresh
- 1 1/2 tablespoons sage fresh
- 1 1/2 tablespoons Paprika
- ½ table spoon of salt
- ½ Table spoon of black pepper
- 1 1/2 large lemon

DIRECTIONS

Wash the chicken and remove any inners and drain the excess water.

Place the unpeeled but scored lemon inside the chicken.

Spread the butter on the outer skin of the chicken evenly.

Add finely chopped rosemary and sage over the skin of the chicken.

Squeeze ½ juice of the lemon over the chicken then leave the remainder of the lemon in the crockpot. Add salt and pepper then finally sprinkle the paprika over the remainder of the chicken.

Cook on low setting 5 1/2 to 6 hours or until cooked.

Duck and Orange Stir-fry

YIELD

SERVES 3-4

PREP TIME 10 MINUTES | **TOTAL TIME** 15 MINUTES

INGREDIENTS

- Fat for cooking Ghee / Coconut oil
- 1 Roasted duck
- 1 Medium sliced onion
- 2 cloves garlic, minced
- 2 tsp. grated ginger
- 1 Tbs. orange zest
- 2/3 cup orange juice
- 1/4 chicken stock
- 3 lb. bok choy leaves
- 1 segmented orange

DIRECTIONS

Pick the meat from the roasted duck and cut the skin in thin slices for garnish at the end. Stir-fry the onion for 3 minutes with some cooking fat.

Add the ginger and garlic and stir-fry for another minute or two. Add the orange juice, zest and stock and bring to a boil. Add the duck to the wok and let the whole preparation simmer for about 3 minutes. Remove the meat from the wok, add the bok choy and cook until just wilted. Serve the duck on a bed of bok choy and garnish with orange segments and crispy duck skin.

Roast Goose with Prune, Apple and Apricot Stuffing

YIELD
SERVES (SEE BELOW)
PREP TIME | TOTAL TIME (SEE BELOW)

9 lb. goose will serve 4-6 people
11 lb. bird will serve 6-8
13 lb. bird 8-9 people
20 minutes per half-kilo/ 1 lb. 2 oz.,

INGREDIENTS

- 1 Goose 9-13 lbs.
- 4 med carrots
- 3/4 - 1 med Onions
- 2-3 Parsnips
- 2 Stalks celery

Depending on the DIRECTIONS used read on

DIRECTIONS

Before roasting, remove any surplus fat from inside the body cavity, then
prick the skin, rub in salt and pepper and brush the goose lightly with oil. Put it, breast side up, on a rack in a roasting tin, to allow the fat to drain off and cover with foil. Alternatively, roast the bird on a bed of root vegetables, such as parsnips, celery, carrots or onions - the fat will fry and caramelize the vegetables, which can be served with the meat or
Puréed for use in a gravy or sauce. Roast the goose in an oven preheated to 180 C / 350 F / Gas 4, allowing around 20 minutes per half-kilo/ 1 lb. 2 oz., Remember to remove the foil for the last 30-40 minutes of cooking.

As with turkeys, the neck end of the goose can be stuffed. - A fruit-based mixture is best to complement the rich meat. If you wish to stuff the body cavity, ensure that it is well washed out beforehand and that the stuffing is properly cooked through before serving. Also don't pack the stuffing in too tightly, or it will be difficult for the heat to penetrate. Red cabbage is a traditional partner to goose, as are roasted winter root vegetables.

1 oven-ready goose, around 11 lb. goes with:

Apple and apricot fruit stuffing:

- 4 oz. stoned prunes, roughly chopped
- 4 oz. dried apricots, roughly chopped
- 3 fl oz. port
- 2 eating apples, peeled, cored and diced
- 1 small red onion, chopped
- Half-teaspoon ground cinnamon
- Quarter-teaspoon ground nutmeg
- Salt and pepper

DIRECTIONS

Mix all the ingredients together, adding just enough egg to bind.

Alternatively Forcemeat Stuffing:

- 1 small onion, chopped
- 1 celery stick, chopped
- The goose liver, finely chopped
- Finely grated zest and juice 1 orange
- 8 oz. good quality pork sausage meat
- 1 teaspoon fresh thyme leaves, or 1 level teaspoon dried thyme
- 3 tablespoons chopped parsley
- 2 oz. ground nuts
- 1 egg, lightly beaten
- Freshly grated nutmeg
- Salt and pepper

DIRECTIONS

Mix all the ingredients together, adding just enough egg to bind.

Alternatively Apple and Quince Sauce:

- 2 quinces, peeled, cored and diced
- 1 1/2 lb. cooking apples, peeled, cored and cut into chunks
- Juice 1 orange
- Generous glass of port
- 1 cinnamon stick

DIRECTIONS

Put the quinces into a pan with just enough water to cover. Now simmer gently for 30-40 minutes until tender. If necessary, boil hard to reduce the water to just a

117

few tablespoons. Add all the remaining sauce ingredients, cover and cook until the apples have collapsed. Serve hot or cold with the goose.

Prepare the fruit and forcemeat stuffing's. Remove the excess fat from inside the goose. Put the forcemeat stuffing into the neck end, pressing it in firmly and then tucking the flap of skin neatly down around it. Secure firmly underneath with a skewer. Put the fruit stuffing into the body cavity. Season the goose and put on a trivet in a roasting tray. Cover and roast in an oven preheated to 350°F until tender, allowing 20-25 minutes per pound, removing the foil for the last 30-40 minutes of cooking. While the goose is cooking, make the applesauce. Serve hot or cold with the goose.

··

Roast Goose with Chestnut Stuffing

YIELD
SERVES 4
PREP TIME 25 MINUTES | **TOTAL TIME** 4-6 HOURS

INGREDIENTS

- 1 leek, sliced
- 1 onion, quartered
- 6kg / 12lb goose, with giblets
- salt and freshly ground pepper to taste
- Goose fat, for roasting
- For the gravy
- goose giblets
- 1 Tbs. arrowroot

For stuffing recipe see: Chestnut Stuffing.

DIRECTIONS

Preheat the oven to 200 C/ 400 F/Gas 4.
Place the leek and onion into the goose cavity.
Prick the skin of the goose all over with a fork and rub in the salt and freshly ground black pepper. Rub a little goose fat over the legs of the goose and cover them well with aluminium foil.

Line a deep roasting dish with more aluminum foil, enough to make a parcel to enclose the goose.

Sit the goose onto a wire rack in the roasting tin and cover with the aluminum foil. Transfer to the oven and roast for about 15 minutes per 450g /16 oz plus an extra 20 minutes.

(This 6 kg/12 lb goose will need approx. 3 1/2 hours.)

After an hour of roasting, remove the foil cover and baste the goose with the juices collected. Check that the legs aren't burning and baste them too. Drain off any excess fat into a separate roasting tray. Return the goose to the oven to cook, repeating the basting every 30 minutes. Return the goose to the oven uncovered for the last 45 minutes of roasting, or until completely cooked through. Test the goose is cooked by piercing the thigh meat with a metal skewer. If the juices run clear, the goose is ready.

Remove from the oven and leave to rest in a warm place for 20 minutes before serving.

For the gravy, place the goose giblets into a large saucepan filled with about 2.6 liters 4 pints of water. Bring to the boil and simmer for three hours, then strain. Return the liquid to the saucepan and simmer. Add the corn flour or arrowroot and stir well to thicken.

To serve, carve the goose and place onto warmed plates. Serve the stuffing alongside with gravy poured over.

....

Poached Partridges
[England, 15ᵗʰ century recipe]

YIELD
SERVES 3-4
PREP TIME 20 MINUTES | **TOTAL TIME** 1-2 HOURS

YIELD
SERVES 3-4
TAKES Approx. 1-2 hours

INGREDIENTS

- 4 Marrow bones
- lb. To 2 1/lb. partridge (or alternatively quail)
- 6 Peppercorns
- Coconut Oil for frying
- 2 1/2 cups Beef stock
- 1   cup grape juice
- 1   cup apple juice
- 1/4 teaspoon Ground cloves
- 1/2 teaspoon Mace
- 1/8 teaspoon Saffron
- 1/2 teaspoon Ginger
- 1 Tbs. fresh chopped Parsley.

DIRECTIONS

Secure the cavities of the bird. Brown it in oil. Add the stock, juice, cloves, and mace. Simmer for 1 1/2 hours, or until tender. Remove the bird, carve, and keep warm. Add the saffron and ginger, simmer the sauce letting it reduce somewhat, until it is well colored by the saffron. Check the seasoning.

Pour the sauce over the bird and sprinkle with freshly chopped parsley, Serve and enjoy.

....

Roast Pheasant

YIELD

SERVES 3-4

PREP TIME 20 MINUTES | **TOTAL TIME** 1-2 HOURS

INGREDIENTS

- 1 2-3 lb. pheasant
- Salt to season
- Freshly ground black pepper
- 1 bay leaf
- 1 clove garlic
- Few celery leaves / 1 slice lemon and 4 slices bacon

DIRECTIONS

Preheat oven to moderate (350 degrees) Sprinkle the pheasant inside and out with salt and pepper. Place the bay leaf, garlic, celery leaves and lemon in the cavity. Tie the legs together with string and turn the wings under.
Cover the breast with bacon. Place the pheasant, breast up, on a rack in a baking pan and roast until tender, about thirty minutes per pound, basting with drippings.

SAUCE:

Remove the pheasant to a warm serving platter and add one cup of broth to the pan. Stir over moderate heat, scraping loose the browned particles.
Blend one tablespoon of arrowroot with just enough water to combine and slowly stir into the gravy. When the gravy is thickened and smooth, add the cooked pheasant liver, finely chopped.

....

Quail and Grapes

YIELD

SERVES 3-4

PREP TIME 20 MINUTES | **TOTAL TIME** 55 MINUTES

INGREDIENTS

- 6 jumbo quail, about 4 to 5 ounces each
- Salt and pepper
- 1 1/2 teaspoons grated garlic
- 6 large rosemary sprigs, plus 1/2 teaspoon chopped
- 6 large thyme sprigs, plus 1/2 teaspoon chopped
- 2 tablespoons olive oil
- 6 small red boiling onions (about 1/2 pound), peeled and quartered
- 1 teaspoon lemon juice
- 1 pound grapes, cut into 6 small clusters

DIRECTIONS

Rinse quail and pat dry. Season inside and out with salt and pepper. Put a small amount of grated garlic in each bird's cavity, as well as the chopped rosemary and thyme. Drizzle birds with 1 tablespoon olive oil, and let marinate at room temperature for at least 1 hour. (You may refrigerate for several hours or overnight; bring to room temperature before roasting.)

Heat oven to 450 degrees. Place onions in a small ovenproof skillet or pie pan, and season with salt and pepper. Toss with lemon juice and remaining 1 tablespoon olive oil to coat. Bake until slightly softened and caramelized, about 10 minutes. Set aside.

Spread remaining rosemary and thyme sprigs on a baking sheet or in a low-sided roasting pan. Lay quail on top of herbs, breast-side down. Roast for about 15 minutes, until puffed and lightly browned. Turn birds breast-side up and surround with roasted onions and grape clusters. Continue roasting for 10 minutes more. If necessary, put birds under the broiler to crisp the skin. Let rest 10 minutes and serve.

....

Holiday Turkey

YIELD
SERVES ...MANY
PREP TIME 25 MINUTES | **TOTAL TIME** 5-6 HOURS

INGREDIENTS
- 1 turkey, size does not matter, but I do prefer a small organic turkey.
- 1 pound non-cured bacon (optional, can be done with or without bacon).
- 1 onion, whole but peeled
- 1 large sprig of fresh rosemary.
- 1 bunch of fresh basil.
- 2-4 bay leaves.
- sea salt and pepper to taste.

DIRECTIONS
After thawing turkey, rinse well in cool water and then pat dry. Place in roasting pan. Stuff peeled onion into turkey with rosemary and basil.
Lightly salt and pepper skin of turkey.
Carefully lift up skin on the breast area, slide 1 or 2 bay leaves under the skin, as

far down as you can without ripping skin, if using 2 on each side, make it about an inch or two apart. Next, wrap the entire top of the turkey in bacon. I just lay mine on top like a lattice. Chris-crossing it.

Cover with roasting pan lid, or foil if no lid.

Bake at 225° F over night. However, I have done it at 325° for 5 hours.

The turkey is so juicy and moist and is oh so easy to take off the bones. If you're doing a chicken, duck or any other small poultry, bake at 325° for 1 1/2 hours.

··

Roast Turkey
(With Olde English Chestnut Stuffing)

YIELD

SERVES ...MANY

PREP TIME 25 MINUTES | **TOTAL TIME** 5-6 HOURS

INGREDIENTS

- 5-6 kg (11-13 lb.) turkey, thawed if frozen
- 3 Tbs. goose fat
- Fresh sage leaves, optional
- 10-12 rashers (slices) streaky bacon
- 1 onion and 1 carrot, peeled and roughly chopped
- 2 sticks celery, chopped
- 8-12 unpeeled shallots
- 18 cocktail sausages

(For stuffing recipe see)
Olde English Chestnut Stuffing

INGREDIENTS

- 8 large, stoned prunes
- 2 Tbs. brandy
- 454g (1 lb.) pack Cumberland style sausages
- 2 rashers dry-cured unsmoked streaky bacon, chopped

- 200g pack cooked and peeled chestnuts, chopped
- 1 cooking apple, peeled, cored and finely chopped
- Finely grated zest and juice of 1 lemon
- 1/2 tsp. grated nutmeg
- Salt and ground black pepper

DIRECTIONS

Pour boiling water over the prunes in a small bowl to cover them. Leave for 20 mins. to plump up. Drain off water, chop prunes, then put them in a larger bowl and add the brandy. Skin sausages and mix the meat with the bacon and chestnuts, apple, zest and juice from half the lemon (keep the shell), nutmeg and seasoning.

Push just over half the stuffing into the neck end of the bird. Secure with 2 bamboo or metal skewers. Spoon the rest of the stuffing into a shallow, greased baking dish and set aside until ready to cook.

For the gravy:

- About 600 ml (1 pint) hot chicken stock.
- 1-2 tsp. corn flour [or arrowroot]
- 100ml (3 1/2 fl oz.) Marsala, Madeira or cherry.

DIRECTIONS

Pull any feathers out of the turkey, with tweezers. Wipe it with kitchen paper. Push just over half the stuffing into the neck end of the bird.

Secure with 2 bamboo or metal skewers. Spoon the rest of the stuffing into a shallow, buttered baking dish and set aside until ready to cook. Weigh turkey and calculate the cooking time about 3 1/2 hours in total

Set the oven to Gas Mark 5 or 190°C (375°F). Rub the other lemon half over the turkey, squeezing out the juice as you go, and put both lemon shells inside the bird. Smear turkey breast and legs with goose fat or butter. Season and season with sage leaves, if you like. Stretch bacon slices with the back of a knife. Overlap them in a lattice over the breast and secure with string. Tie the legs together.

Put the bird in a large roasting tin, with the neck and heart pushed underneath the stuffed neck end, to keep it in shape. Roast, basting now and then with the cooking juices. After 1 hour, add the onion, carrot, celery and shallots to the tin and cover the whole tin with foil. Cook for another 2-2 1/2 hours, checking hourly. Take out shallots when they are cooked and set aside.

Check the turkey is cooked by inserting a skewer into the thickest part of the thigh. The juices should run clear. If not, cook for another 15 mins, then test again. Put the bird on a warm serving platter, cover with foil and keep in a warm place for 20-30 mins. before carving.

Put the sausages in a small roasting tin, along with the dish of stuffing, and cook in the oven for 25-30 mins.

To make the gravy: Transfer the onion, carrot and celery from the roasting tin to a pan, and pour the juices into a large jug, scraping all the crunchy bits from the tin into the pan. Leave cooking juices for 5-10 mins to settle,

Pour off the fat into a small bowl. Add the juices to the pan along with some chicken stock and simmer for 10-15 mins until the vegetables are soft. Now mash the vegetables in the pan. Mix the corn flour with the fortified wine and whisk into the gravy. Boil for a few minutes until thickened. Strain into a jug, now pour into your gravy boat.

Garnish your turkey with bay leaves, if you like. Serve with the sausages, shallots and gravy.

Oven-Baked Carrot Fries

YIELD

SERVES 4

PREP TIME 5 MINUTES | **TOTAL TIME** 25 MINUTES

INGREDIENTS

- 1 1/2 pounds carrots (10 medium)
- 2 tablespoons olive oil
- 2 teaspoons finely chopped fresh rosemary
- 1/2 teaspoon salt
- Pinch of freshly ground pepper

DIRECTIONS

Preheat an oven to 425°F. Line a jellyroll pan with aluminum foil.

Cut away the tip and end of each carrot. Peel the carrots if desired.

Cut a carrot in half crosswise. Next, cut each half in half lengthwise.

Finally, cut each half in half lengthwise again. You will end up with 8 sticks from the carrot. Repeat with the other carrots.

In a large bowl, combine the carrot sticks, olive oil, rosemary, salt and pepper. Stir with a rubber spatula until the carrot sticks are evenly coated with all the other ingredients.

Dump the carrots onto the foil-lined pan, scraping out any herbs that are clinging to the sides of the bowl. Spread the sticks out as much as possible.

Bake until the carrots are tender and well browned, about 20 minutes.

Remove the pan from the oven. Serve the carrot fries hot or at room temperature.

....

Sweet Potato Chips

YIELD

SERVES 3-4

PREP TIME 5 MINUTES | **TOTAL TIME** 45 MINUTES

INGREDIENTS

- 2-3 sweet potatoes, peeled and sliced
- 1/4 cup oil
- cayenne pepper

METHOD

Peel and slice the sweet potatoes. In a small bowl, sprinkle the Cayenne Pepper into the ¼ cup of oil and blend. In medium bowl, add the oil blend to the potato and stir until each slice is lightly coated.

Spread slices in 10" x 15.5" stoneware pan and bake at 400°F for 30-40 minutes or until edges brown and crisp, turning/stirring every 10-15 minutes. (If you use a metal pan, it may take longer to bake to desired crispiness.) If desired, salt after baking. ENJOY!

CHAPTER 12

BEEF

Italian-Style Roast Beef

YIELD

SERVES 10-12

PREP TIME 25 MINUTES | **TOTAL TIME** 21/2 HOURS

INGREDIENTS

- 4-pound bottom round roast beef.
- 2 large onions, sliced
- 3 cloves garlic, chopped
- 1 tablespoon garlic powder,
- 1 tablespoon oregano, plus more to taste
- 2 cups fresh baby carrots

DIRECTIONS

In Dutch oven, sear sides of roast over high heat until well browned.
[Brown extensively to seal in the juices. Brown in a few Tbs. of oil in the dutch oven on medium high heat, on all sides.] Remove from pan and set aside. Lower heat to medium and add onion and garlic, cooking about 3 minutes until softened.

Season meat with garlic powder and oregano then return to pan. Add one cup cold water to pan. Cover and cook on medium-low heat for about 3 1/2 hours. Add more water as needed to create a rich au jus. After the second hour, arrange baby carrots around the meat, seasoning with garlic powder and oregano to taste. When meat is tender, remove from meat, carrots and onions from pan. Put meat on a carving board and slice; place carrots in serving bowl with cooked onion.

Bacon Stuffed Flank Steak

YIELD

SERVES 3-4

PREP TIME 10 MINUTES | **TOTAL TIME** 55 MINUTES

INGREDIENTS

- 1 1/2 lbs. flank steaks, trimmed and pounded evenly to 1/2 inch thickness
- 1 teaspoon garlic salt
- pepper
- 8-10 slices bacon, cooked
- 2 tablespoons chopped parsley
- 1 onion, sliced
- 1/2 lb. mushroom, sliced (about 8-12)

DIRECTIONS

Preheat broiler or prepare barbecue.

Season steak with garlic salt and pepper.

Score steak diagonally twice, reversing direction creating "x" s or Chris-cross pattern.

Place bacon lengthwise over steak and sprinkle with parsley.

Roll steak lengthwise, securing with toothpicks at 1-inch intervals.
Broil or grill, turning frequently until browned on all sides and cooked to degree of doneness desired (20 minutes for med rare).

While steak is grilling/broiling, cook mushroom and onion slices in bacon grease in same skillet for 15-20 minutes or until browned to desired browning.

When steak is done remove toothpicks and cut meat into eight 1-inch rounds and top with mushroom and onion slices.

Swiss Steak

YIELD

SERVES 3-4

PREP TIME 10 | **TOTAL TIME** 3-4 HOURS

INGREDIENTS

- 1 inch slice of Swiss steak or top round
- 1 can V-8 juice
- 1-2 Tbs. honey
- Coconut /Avocado oil
- pepper to taste

DIRECTIONS

Brown steak in hot skillet on both sides in coconut / avocado oil. Remove steak from skillet and add 1 can of V-8 juice, honey and pepper. Heat until hot and the steak leavings are mixed into sauce. Place the steak in a dutch oven with lid. Pour on sauce, cover and place in oven at 375 F. Bake for 3 hours and then uncover. Bake another hour or until sauce is cooked down and thick.

Meat should be fork tender. The sauce is wonderful over sautéed zucchini, summer squash, and onions.

Pepper Steak

YIELD

SERVES 2-3

PREP TIME 5 MINUTES | **TOTAL TIME** 20 MINUTES

INGREDIENTS

- 1 pound round steak cut 1/2 inch thick
- 2 Tbs. olive oil
- 1 medium onion, sliced
- 1 medium green pepper, sliced
- dash garlic salt

- 1/4 cup water
- 2 cups shredded carrots (about 4 medium carrots)

DIRECTIONS

Cut meat in half lengthwise with a sharp knife, then crosswise into thin slices. Brown meat in hot oil, then add onion and pepper; cook 1 to 2 minutes. Stir in water, sprinkle on garlic salt, and cook about 5 minutes, stirring constantly. Serve on a bed of carrots.

Peppered Beef Tenderloin

YIELD

SERVES 10

PREP TIME 15 MINUTES | **TOTAL TIME** 55 MINUTES

INGREDIENTS

- 1 Tbs. Pepper; coarsely ground
- 1 1/2 tsp. Fennel seeds; crushed
- 1/2 tsp. Red pepper; ground
- 1/8 tsp. Nutmeg; ground
- 1/8 tsp. Mustard; dry
- 1/8 tsp. Garlic powder
- 1/8 tsp. Onion powder
- 5 lb. Beef tenderloin (Adjust according to servings)

DIRECTIONS

Combine spices in a small bowl; set aside. Trim fat from tenderloin; rub with pepper mixture. Place tenderloin on a rack coated with cooking spray; place rack on a broiler pan. Insert meat thermometer into thickest portion of meat. Bake at 375F for 50 minutes or until thermometer registers 140* (rare). Place tenderloin on serving platter; cover and let stand 10 minutes. Cut into thin slices.

Grilled Steak with Provincial Herbs

YIELD

SERVES 4-5
PREP TIME 5 MINUTES | **TOTAL TIME** 12 MINUTES*

INGREDIENTS

- 4 - Natural grass fed Gourmet Steaks
- 1 Tbs. Olive oil
- 2 Garlic cloves, minced
- 2 tsp. minced fresh rosemary or 1 tsp. dried, crumbled
- 2 tsp. minced fresh thyme or 1 tsp. dried, crumbled
- 2 tsp. minced fresh basil or 1 tsp. dried, crumbled
- Fresh ground pepper

DIRECTIONS

Place the steaks in a shallow dish. Rub both sides with oil, garlic and herbs. Add pepper. Let them stand 1 hour *.
Prepare barbeque (high heat) or preheat broiler. Cook steaks 2 inches from heat source to desired taste, 4 minutes per side for rare.

···

Paleo-Chili

YIELD

SERVES 4-5
PREP TIME 25 MINUTES | **TOTAL TIME** 4 HOURS

INGREDIENTS

- 2 lbs. ground buffalo
- 1 cup chopped onion
- 3 cloves chopped garlic
- 2-4 Tbs fat (I use pork fat)
- 2 cups canned chopped tomatoes
- 4 Tablespoons chili powder.

- 1 teaspoon dry oregano
- 1 teaspoon ground cumin
- 1 teaspoon salt
- 1 cup water

DIRECTIONS

Brown ground buffalo with chopped onion and chopped garlic, in fat. Then add chopped tomatoes, chili powder, oregano, cumin, and salt.

Add water, then simmer the mixture for at least two hours, until the meat is very tender and the tomatoes pretty much cook into the sauce.

Slow cook for four hours is not too much, but check to make sure it does not go dry.

Bison Chili

YIELD

SERVES 4-5

PREP TIME 15 MINUTES | **TOTAL TIME** 65 MINUTES

INGREDIENTS

- 1 Tablespoon coconut oil
- 1 3/4 lbs. ground bison
- 1/2 onion, chopped
- 2 1/2 cups chopped celery
- 2 cloves garlic
- 1 12 oz. jar Organic salsa. (I recommend you make it yourself. It's Simple. garlic, Fresh tomato, red pepper, green pepper, salt pepper) *
- 1 8 oz. can of tomatoes
- 2 tsp. cumin
- 2 tsp. chili powder
- 2 tsp. thyme leaves
- 2 tsp. sea salt

DIRECTIONS

First sauté (medium heat) the onion, celery and garlic until onions are translucent about 3 or 4 minutes. Then you add the meat, cumin, thyme, and chili powder. Stir while this cooks for about 5 to 6 minutes. Then dump in the salsa, tomatoes and salt. I also added about a 1/4 cup of mild green chili's.
Then let this simmer for at least an hour.

Paleo Chili Texas

YIELD

SERVES 3-4

PREP TIME 15 MINUTES | **TOTAL TIME** 130 MINUTES

"This legendary food, named "the state dish of Texas" by the Texans legislature, has been a source of many debates, both as to the origin and the correct ingredients. It has been said by some of the most respected figures in the chili world that 'anyone who would put beans in chili doesn't know beans about chili.' The following recipe is a "no frills" version. Included are a couple of the most common variations for the more adventurous who would "fly in the face" of Texas tradition."

INGREDIENTS

- 2 ounces animal fat (beef suet or uncured bacon)
- 2 pounds coarsely ground beef
- 1/2 cup finely chopped onion
- 2 cloves garlic, minced
- 2 tablespoons chili powder, or more if desired
- 1/2 teaspoon ground cumin
- 1/8 teaspoon dried oregano (optional)
- Salt to taste

DIRECTIONS

In a large skillet (preferably cast-iron), render fat over medium heat and remove rinds. Add ground beef to skillet and cook until just brown. Add onion and garlic.
Add chili powder, cumin, and oregano, and mix well. Add salt conservatively. Reduce heat to low and let simmer for at least 2 hours. The texture and flavor will change greatly as all of the ingredients blend together. Add water as needed during cooking, keeping in mind that the final product should be somewhat thick.

English Cottage Pie Filling

YIELD

SERVES 4-5

PREP TIME 15 MINUTES | **TOTAL TIME** 45 MINUTES

INGREDIENTS

- Virgin Olive oil
- 1 1/2 cups chopped onion
- 1/2 cup chopped carrot
- 1 (8-ounce) package cremini or button mushrooms, sliced
- 1 pound extra-lean ground beef
- 2 tablespoons no-salt-added organic tomato paste
- 1 cup lower-sodium paleo beef broth
- 1/4 teaspoon freshly ground black pepper
- 1/4 cup chopped fresh parsley
- 1 tablespoon fresh thyme leaves
- 1/2 teaspoon salt

DIRECTIONS

Heat the oil in a large nonstick skillet over medium-high heat. Add the onion and carrot sauté 5 minutes. Add mushrooms; sauté for 5 minutes or until lightly browned. Remove vegetables from skillet. Add beef to pan; cook 5 minutes or until browned, stirring to crumble. Stir in tomato paste, and cook 3 minutes. Stir in broth and pepper. Return vegetables to pan, and a simmer. Stir in parsley, thyme, and salt.

....

Bobotie

(Bobotie is a South African beef casserole, traditionally made with bread and milk.)
This recipe is inspired by the original dish but modified for Paleo

YIELD

SERVES 4-5

INGREDIENTS

- 2 lbs. ground beef
- 2 medium sized onions, 1/4" dice
- 2 Teaspoon olive oil / Coconut oil.
- 2 Teaspoons curry powder (or more if you like it spicy)
- 1 Teaspoon turmeric
- 2 Teaspoon lemon juice
- 1/2 Teaspoon black pepper
- 2 Cup purple cabbage, finely chopped
- 2 large eggs
- 1/2 Cup mixed dried berries (raisons, currant, cranberry)
- 1/2 Cup crab apples, finely chopped
- 2 bay leaves, crushed with mortar and pestle
- 1/2 C raw almonds

DIRECTIONS

Preheat oven to 350F. Fry onions in the oil over medium heat until golden colored. Add the curry powder and turmeric. Fry for two minutes stirring all the time, then add the lemon juice, salt and pepper.

In the meanwhile, crumble the ground meat into a pan and cook over medium-low heat until mostly done.

Mix the meat, cabbage, onion mixture and fruit with 1 egg. Pack into a casserole dish and sprinkle with the crushed bay leaves.

Pulse the almonds in a blender on high until coarsely ground, then mix with the remaining egg. Spread this mixture out on top of the meat to make a thin almond crust.

Bake uncovered for 30 minutes.

Paleo Beef Curry

YIELD

SERVES 2-4
PREP TIME 20 MINUTES | **TOTAL TIME** 80 MINUTES

INGREDIENTS

- 2 Tablespoons coconut oil
- 1 cup chopped onion
- 1 cup chopped celery
- 3 cloves garlic
- 450g diced beef
- 400ml canned diced tomatoes
- 250ml salsa (I made mine fresh with 1 cup of green peppers, 5 cherry
-     tomatoes and 3 olives)
- 1 teaspoon cumin powder
- 1 Tablespoon chili powder
- 1 t ground thyme

DIRECTIONS

Heat coconut oil in a large frying pan, then sauté the celery, onion and garlic for 3 minutes, until the onion is translucent.
Add meat and spice, stirring well, and cook for 5 minutes.

Add tomatoes and salsa, stir well, and then simmer for at least an hour.

Superb served over riced cauliflower, topped with flaked almonds.

....

Trinidad Inspired East Indian Beef Curry

YIELD

SERVES 4-5

INGREDIENTS

- 1 1/2 lb. beef, cut into cubes (trim off excess fat)
- 2 large onion
- 1 inch piece ginger root
- 3 cloves garlic
- 2 green chili peppers
- 3 tablespoons oil
- 4 tablespoons curry powder
- salt, pepper to taste
- 2 1/2 cups coconut milk

DIRECTIONS

1) Finely chop onions, ginger root and garlic, remove stalks and seeds from chili peppers and chop finely too.

2) Heat oil in heavy pot, add the chopped ingredients and stir fry until light brown.

3) Add curry powder and continue frying for a few min more (may have to add a little water so that the spices will not burn).

4) Add meat and continue stirring until it is well browned and coated with the spice mixture.

5) Add salt and pepper to taste and continue stirring.

6) Add coconut milk, stir thoroughly, then reduce heat and cover pot. Cook on low until meat is tender (about 1 1/4 hours).

7) Adjust seasonings, if necessary. Can be served with Mango Chutney.

Pork Curry- Prepare same way.
Chicken Curry- prepare the same way- but with less cooking time.
Shrimp Curry- prepare same way- Note shrimp cook time less.

Curry Hot Pot

YIELD

SERVES 4-5

PREP TIME 15 MINUTES | **TOTAL TIME** 55 MINUTES

INGREDIENTS

- 1 1/2 lbs. boned chuck
- 2 Tbs. olive oil Coconut oil
- 2 med. onions, sliced
- 1 apple, peeled and cubed
- 1 Tbs. curry powder
- 2 tomatoes, chopped
- 1/4 cup raisins
- 2 cups beef broth
- 1/4 tsp. pepper
- 1 Tbs. honey

DIRECTIONS

Cut chuck lengthwise into 1 1/2 inch strips and crosswise into thin slices.
Brown in hot oil. Add onions, apple and curry, and sauté. Stir in tomatoes, raisins, beef broth, pepper, and honey. Bring to a boil. Simmer covered for 40 minutes, or until the meat is tender.

Beef heart

YIELD

SERVES 2-3

PREP TIME 20 MINUTES | **TOTAL TIME** 2 HOURS

INGREDIENTS

- One beef heart
- Fresh ground pepper, about 1/4 cup
- 4 large onions, sliced as thinly as possible.
- 2 garlic cloves very finely diced
- Shallow pan large enough to hold the heart

DIRECTIONS

Oven pre-heated to 250F. Mix the garlic and pepper together. Using a sharp knife, cut down into the heart about 1". Carefully cut in a spiral towards the center keeping the cuts 1" apart. Lay the heart out in one long strip.
Spread the pepper/garlic mix evenly over the meat. It will be a very thin
layer and does not have to coat the entire heart. The idea is to not have any clumps of the mix. Evenly layer the thinly sliced onion on the heart. Roll the heart back together, jelly roll fashion. Secure with twine.

Put the heart into the shallow pan and put into the oven. Using a meat thermometer to determine internal temperature, cook until: Rare (red center) - 110F Med rare (still red center, but shading towards pint) - 120F Med (pink center) - 135F Med Well (a little pink in the center) - 145F Well Done (no pink at all) - 160F.
When internal temperature reaches desired level, remove from oven and cover lightly with foil. The heat in the center will continue to rise for another 5 mins. Cooking times will be determined by the size of the heart.

Primal Tongue

YIELD

SERVES 8-10

PREP TIME 20 MINUTES | **TOTAL TIME** 3 HOURS

INGREDIENTS

- 1-3 lb. large beef tongue
- 1 Onion, quartered
- 1 Carrot, sliced
- 3 Ribs of leafy celery
- 6 Sprigs of parsley
- 2 Bay leaves
- 10 Peppercorns, cracked
- 1 Dried chili, optional

All are tasty. They can be purchased fresh, smoked and pickled. The most desired, in order of preference, are: calf, lamb, beef and pork.

DIRECTIONS

To prepare: scrub the tongue well. Add all the ingredients in water and bring to boil Immerse the tongue in seasoned boiling water to cover, reduce heat and simmer gently for at least one hour. Up to 3 hours for large beef tongues.

Then drain, plunge into cold water to cool the meat enough to handle, skin it, and trim any bones and gristle from the root. Finally, return it to the cooking water to re-heat it before serving. Alternatively, chill entirely and serve as a cold cut. To carve, start by cutting through the hump parallel to the base, but towards the tip cut diagonally for better looking presentation.

....

Fritada

YIELD

SERVES 8-10

PREP TIME 15 MINUTES | **TOTAL TIME** 60 MINUTES

INGREDIENTS

- One medium onion
- Salt and pepper
- Blood from the animal
- 6 cloves garlic
- Small and large intestines
- Heart
- Liver
- Pancreas

DIRECTIONS

Open and scrub intestines with coconut or olive oil. Wash with boiling water, vinegar and salt. Wash liver and remove skin. Chop into small pieces. Cook all ingredients except the blood. When meat is cooked,
then add blood and stir. Add 1 cup cold water.

This dish is unbelievably delicious.

At a fiesta, with 20 or so cooks, the cooks eat all the fritada while working, leaving none for the attendees who arrive later!
It's their payment for their work.

Roast Lamb with Herbs

YIELD

SERVES 3-4

PREP TIME 20 MINUTES | **TOTAL TIME** 1-3 HOURS

INGREDIENTS

- 1 garlic clove, minced
- 1 tsp. pepper
- 1 crushed bay leaf
- 1/2 tsp. ginger
- 1/2 tsp. marjoram
- 1/2 tsp. thyme
- 1/2 tsp. sage
- 1 Tbs. oil
- 1 leg of lamb

DIRECTIONS

Mix garlic, seasonings, herbs and oil together. Rub on the roast. Place lamb on rack in roasting pan. Cook, uncovered, at 300F for approx. 30 minutes per lb.

Boneless Lamb Shoulder Roast

YIELD

SERVES 3-4

PREP TIME 20 MINUTES | **TOTAL TIME** 2 HOURS

INGREDIENTS

- 1 cup parsley leaves

- 4 medium cloves garlic
- salt and freshly ground black pepper
- about 2 Tbs. extra virgin olive oil
- 1 boned lamb shoulder (3-4 pound), trimmed of surface fat

DIRECTIONS

Preheat oven to 300 F. Mince the garlic and parsley together until quite fine. Add a big pinch of salt, some pepper and enough olive oil to make it slurry. Smear this onto and into the lamb, making sure to get it into every nook and cranny possible. Put lamb into a roasting pan lined with foil.

Roast for about 1 1/2 hours, basting with pan juices every 30 minutes or so. When the internal temperature reaches 140 F, turn heat to 400 F and roast about 10 minutes more, until internal temperature is 150 F and the exterior has browned nicely. Let roast sit for about 10 minutes, then carve and serve with some if its juices.

···

Lamb Chops Stuffed with Chicken Livers

YIELD

SERVES 5-6

PREP TIME 15 MINUTES | **TOTAL TIME** 40 MINUTES

INGREDIENTS

- 6 chicken livers, chopped
- 1/2 lb. mushrooms, chopped
- 5 Tbs olive oil
- pepper
- 1 Tbs parsley, finely chopped
- 6 double rib lamb chops

DIRECTIONS

Sauté the livers and mushrooms in 2 Tbs. coconut oil, do not let them brown. Season with pepper Add the parsley. Trim fat from chops and slit them to make pockets. Stuff the pockets with the liver mixture. Heat the remaining oil in heavy casserole, add chops and sear them over high heat in both sides. Cover casserole and bake at 350F for 25 minutes or until tender.

You can skewer chops to close pockets and broil on both sides until cooked. Put chops on a platter, then pour pan juice over them, and serve.

....

Lamb Meatballs Spanish inspired

YIELD
SERVES 2-4
PREP TIME 15 MINUTES | **TOTAL TIME** 40 MINUTES

INGREDIENTS

These little lamb meatballs are dry fried, then cooked in a tasty tomato sauce for an easy to make meal with a Spanish flavor.

- 150 g (5 1/2 oz.) minced lamb
- 1 small onion, chopped finely
- 1 garlic clove, crushed
- 2 teaspoons mixed dried herbs
- 1 small egg white, beaten lightly
- 2 tablespoons brandy
- 100 g (3 1/2 oz.) button mushrooms, sliced
- 300 ml (10 fl oz.) passata (or a 400 g can of chopped tomatoes)
- 1 tablespoon tomato puree
- 1 teaspoon paprika
- 150 ml (5 fl oz.) vegetable stock
- salt and freshly ground black pepper
- chopped fresh parsley to garnish

DIRECTIONS

In a mixing bowl, combine the minced lamb, onion, garlic, dried herbs and egg white. Lightly season with salt and pepper.
Using clean hands, form the mixture into small meatballs.1-2" diameter.

Heat a large non-stick frying pan and add the meatballs, dry frying them until they are lightly browned. Pour in the brandy and let it bubble up for a few moments, and then add the mushrooms, passata, tomato puree, paprika and stock. Heat until simmering, and then cook gently for 20-25 minutes to reduce the liquid by about one third, stirring occasionally.

Garnish with plenty of chopped fresh parsley.

··

Lamb Stew

YIELD
SERVES 2-4
PREP TIME 15 MINUTES | **TOTAL TIME** 45 MINUTES

INGREDIENTS
All done in a frying pan on medium heat.

- 2-3 lbs. lamb, Non trimmed and cubed
- 2 cloves garlic, minced
- 1 teaspoon coconut oil in frying pan
- 1 onion
- 1 cup hot water
- 2/3 large carrots cut into chunks
- Add Broccoli, carrot or other vegetables you desire.
- 1 Tablespoon dried rosemary
- 1 Tablespoon dried thyme
- 1 teaspoon of Salt and Pepper

DIRECTIONS
While onion is frying lightly, cut up lamb steak in cubes. Fry lamb with onion.
1 cup hot water - pour over lamb.
Cover frying pan and simmer.
Slice carrots, put in fry pan and simmer 10 minutes.
Put in pieces of broccoli, or whatever vegetables you are able to eat.
Season with salt and pepper, Fresh rosemary and Thyme.
Cook until tender (about 20-25 minutes)

Lamb Curry

YIELD

SERVES 4-5

PREP TIME 15 MINUTES | **TOTAL TIME** 75 MINUTES*

INGREDIENTS

- 3 lbs. lamb shoulder, trimmed and cubed
- 2 cloves garlic, minced
- 4 onions, sliced
- 1 teaspoon Coconut oil
- 3 tablespoon curry powder
- 2 lemons, sliced
- 4 tablespoon raisins
- 3 apples, peeled, cored, and chopped

DIRECTIONS

Sauté garlic and onions in oil until onions are golden. Sauté lamb cubes 10 minutes, stirring. Add curry powder and onion/garlic to lamb, simmer 5 minutes. Add remaining ingredients. Pour 3 cups of water over all, and bring to a boil. Reduce heat, cover and simmer mixture 1 hour. Best if made 1 day ahead, chilled and then reheated.*

....

Hot Lamb Curry

YIELD

SERVES 4-6

PREP TIME 15 MINUTES | **TOTAL TIME** 1 HOUR 45 MINUTES

INGREDIENTS

- 1.5 lb. boneless lamb cut into 2 inch cubes
- 8 dried red chili's
- 4 Tbs. fat (ghee, coconut oil or lard)
- 1 finely chopped onion

- 6 cloves garlic chopped
- 2 inch piece ginger root finely chopped
- 1 tsp. cumin seeds freshly ground
- 1 tsp. coriander seeds freshly ground
- 1 tsp. fenugreek seeds freshly ground
- 1 tsp. garam masala
- 14 oz. can tomatoes
- 2 Tbs. tomato paste

DIRECTIONS

Chop 4 chili's. Leave the other 4 whole. Heat half the fat in pan, then add garlic ginger and onion. Stir over medium heat until golden. Stir in spices. Cook over medium heat 10 minutes. Stir in tomatoes, paste and chili's. Bring to a gentle boil. Cook over low heat 10 minutes. Meanwhile heat remaining fat in ovenproof pan and cook meat until evenly sealed.

Transfer sauce to meat pan, cover and cook in a 350F oven for 1 1/2 hours until tender.

Lamb Roast Slow Cooker

YIELD

SERVES 4-6

PREP TIME 20 MINUTES | **TOTAL TIME** 5-6 HOURS

INGREDIENTS

- 2 lb. grass fed lamb arm roast
- 1/2 teaspoon salt
- 1 Tablespoon dried rosemary
- 1 Tablespoon dried thyme
- 1/4 teaspoon black pepper
- 5 cloves garlic, halved
- 1 tablespoon coconut oil, as needed
- 1/4 cup Marsala cooking wine

DIRECTIONS

Combine salt, rosemary and black pepper in a small bowl.
Using a sharp knife, make small slits all around the lamb roast and stuff
each slit with a garlic half. Rub the herb mixture all over the roast.
- Pan sear the roast on all sides. Remove from heat.
- Add the coconut oil to the slow cooker pot. Place the roast inside and pour the
wine over it.
Now Cook at low temperature for 5-6 hours.

Irish Lamb Stew – Crockpot Recipe

YIELD

SERVES 4-6

PREP TIME 20 MINUTES | **TOTAL TIME** 5-6 HOURS

INGREDIENTS

- 1-2 pounds lamb, cut up (or broth, bones and leftovers from other recipe)
- 3-4 yellow onions, cut into 1/2" pieces.
- 6-8 carrots, cut into 1/2" slices
- 3-4 cloves garlic, chopped
- 1-2 bay leaves
- 1/2-1 t. dried tarragon
- 1/2-1 t. ground black pepper

DIRECTIONS

Combine the above ingredients in a crockpot with enough water to barely cover. Cook overnight on low (slower cooking lets the veggies flavor through without getting mushy). Allow to cool in order to easily remove the excess fat, the bones, and the bay leaves. Reheat to serve.

CHAPTER 14

PORK

Pork With Rosemary

YIELD
SERVES 4
PREP TIME 20 MINUTES | **TOTAL TIME** 30 MINUTES

INGREDIENTS

- 4 butterfly pork chops
- 1/3 cup organic extra virgin olive oil
- about 2 tablespoons dried, crushed rosemary
- salt and pepper to taste

DIRECTIONS

Marinate pork chops in oil and spices for one hour in the refrigerator. Sauté in a heavy skillet pan over medium heat. Then place in oven for 7-10 minutes until cooked.

Serve with a mixed green salad with a red wine vinaigrette, Mashed, garlic-infused chestnuts are a great accompaniment.

Herbed Pork Roast

YIELD

SERVES 4-6

PREP TIME 25 MINUTES | **TOTAL TIME** 6 HOURS

INGREDIENTS

- 3 pounds pork roast or tenderloin
- 1/2 teaspoon thyme
- 1/2 teaspoon sage
- 1 1/2 teaspoon rosemary
- 1 bay leaf
- 2 fresh leaves basil
- 1 apple, cored, and cut into quarters
- Salt and pepper

DIRECTIONS

Place roast in crock-pot. Cover just to top with water. Add thyme, sage, rosemary, bay leaf, basil, and apple. Add salt and pepper, to taste. Cover, and cook on med. for 5-6 hrs. Note that some people find this recipe bland.

Bacon-Wrapped Pork Tenderloin

YIELD

SERVES 4-6

PREP TIME 20 MINUTES | **TOTAL TIME** 70 MINUTES

INGREDIENTS

Juicy pork tenderloin meets crispy bacon and savoury-sweet apples. Simple enough for a weeknight, but impressive enough for a dinner party too.

- 1 (1-pound) pork tenderloin
- 4 teaspoons olive oil
- 4 to 5 slices thin-cut bacon (about 4 ounces)
- 2 pounds Pink Lady apples, or other firm, sweet apples

- 1 teaspoon kosher salt, plus more for seasoning the tenderloin
- Fresh ground black pepper

DIRECTIONS

Heat the oven to 500°F and arrange a rack at the top.

Coat the tenderloin with 1 teaspoon of the olive oil and season with salt and a generous amount pepper. Wrap the bacon around the tenderloin in a spiral so it completely covers the meat. Place on a baking sheet and roast until the bacon just begins to render, about 10 minutes.

Meanwhile, core the apples, slice into 6 wedges each, and place in a large bowl. Add the remaining 3 teaspoons olive oil, measured salt, and pepper. Toss until well coated.

Scatter the apples around the tenderloin without allowing them to touch each other or the pork, and roast until the bacon is light brown, the underside of the tenderloin is browned and the meat registers 150°F on the underside, and the apples are knife tender, about 10 minutes more.
Set the oven to broil and cook the tenderloin until the apples begin to brown, the bacon is golden brown, and the pork reaches 155°F to 160°F. Let rest at least 5 minutes before serving.

SEAFOOD SHRIMP RECIPES IN COCONUT SAUCE

OMG DELICIOUS RECIPES...ENJOY!

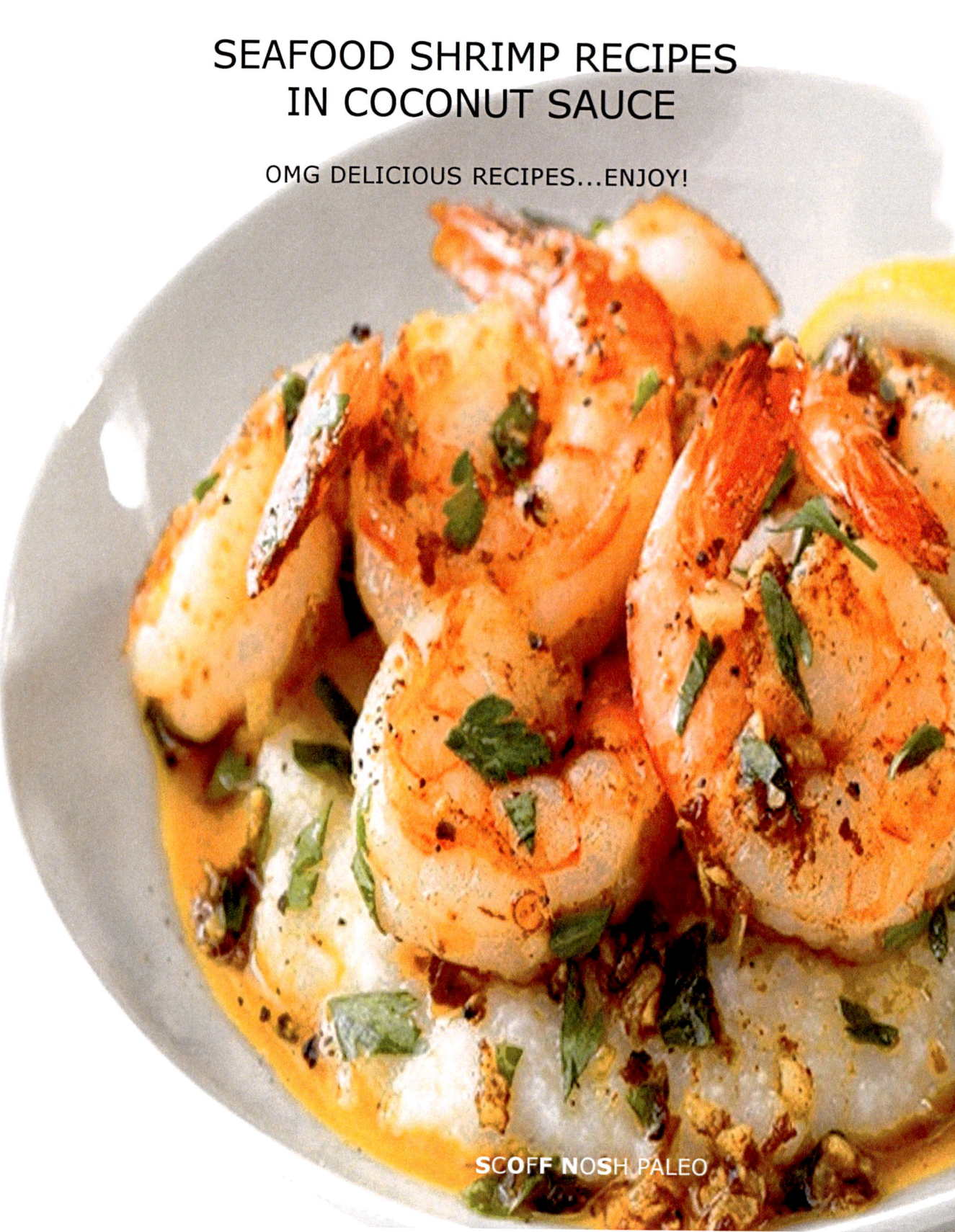

SCOFF NOSH PALEO

CHAPTER 15

SEAFOOD PALEO RECIPES

This being my favorite food by far, living most my life on the East and West Coasts of England I have been privileged to enjoy the amazing taste of fresh caught wild seafood. For the Paleo diet, we ideally only want to eat wild caught fish and seafood to ensure the most natural, healthy and amazing taste.

Shrimp Curry

YIELD

SERVES 4

PREP TIME 15 MINUTES | **TOTAL TIME** 25 MINUTES

INGREDIENTS

- 2 Tbs. olive oil
- 1 medium onion, finely chopped
- 1 (8 oz.) can tomato sauce
- 2 tsp. minced fresh ginger (essential)
- 2 cloves garlic, minced
- 1/2 tsp. cumin
- 1/2 tsp. coriander
- 1/2 tsp. turmeric
- lime juice
- 1 package (6 oz.) frozen shelled, deveined shrimp, thawed.

DIRECTIONS

Heat the oil and sauté onion at low temperature until golden brown. Add tomato sauce, ginger, garlic, and spices. Bring to simmer. Add some water if too thick. Add shrimp to sauce. Simmer 5 minutes. Add some lime juice just before serving.

Shrimp Stuffed Avocado

YIELD

SERVES 4

PREP TIME 10 MINUTES | **TOTAL TIME** 25 MINUTES

INGREDIENTS

- 4-5 avocados, halved, pitted and peeled
- 1lb medium sized cooked shrimp
- 1/2 medium red onion, diced finely
- 2 radishes, diced finely
- 1/2 red bell pepper, diced finely
- 2 celery stalks, diced finely
- 2 hardboiled eggs, diced
- 5 Tablespoons cilantro aioli or paleo mayonnaise
- Juice from 1 lime
- Salt and pepper to taste

DIRECTIONS

Chop shrimp in half, if desired keep a few to garnish. In a medium bowl, combine diced onions, radishes, bell pepper, celery, eggs, shrimp, 1/2 of the lime juice and aioli; mix well. Taste with salt and pepper if necessary.

Drizzle the remaining lime juice over the avocados, this helps keep them from darkening too quickly. Use a spoon to stuff the avocados with shrimp salad filling.

Add any garnishes and serve immediately. Suggestions: Serve with aji or hot sauce to add spice. Also, cilantro aioli served as a salad

Shrimp in Spicy Coconut Sauce

YIELD

SERVES 4-6

PREP TIME 14 MINUTES | **TOTAL TIME** 35 MINUTES

INGREDIENTS

- 1/2 medium red bell pepper, seeded and hopped. *(For the red pepper paste)
- 5 medium shallots, peeled and chopped
- 5 garlic cloves chopped
- 1 inch piece of fresh ginger chopped
- 8 raw macadamia nuts chopped
- 1/4 cup roasted curry powder
- Water as needed

For the sauce:

- 5 tablespoons olive oil
- 1 teaspoon whole black (brown) or yellow mustard seed
- 15 to 20 fresh curry leaves
- Red pepper paste (see above) *
- 1 3/4 cup of water
- 3/4 to 1 teaspoon salt, or to taste
- 1 tablespoon thick tamarind paste.

Finishing the dish:

- 2 pounds medium shrimp.
- 14-ounce can of coconut milk.
- 3 whole fresh hot green chili's

DIRECTIONS

Preparing Red Pepper Paste: Put red pepper, shallots, garlic and ginger into blender in order listed so more moist ingredients are on bottom. Blend and pulse until a paste is made, adding 1-3 tablespoons of water to make a smooth puree. Add cashews and curry powder and puree again to a paste.

Preparing the sauce: Set pan over moderately high heat, add the oil and heat until very hot and almost smoking, then add mustard seeds, the oil should be hot

157

enough for the seeds to "Pop!" As soon as they pop, just a second or two, add the curry leaves. Stir quickly and add the red pepper paste.

Fry, stirring the whole time until paste is reduced, turns red-brown in color and starts to separate from the oil - 7 to 10 minutes. Stir in water, salt and tamarind paste, and bring to boil. Lower heat to low and boil slowly for 4-5 minutes. Strain through a sieve into a bow, pushing out the sauce. Return it to the pan. You can make this in the morning, but use it that day!

Shrimp: Peel and devein shrimp, wash and pat dry. Bring sauce to a gentle simmer. Stir up the coconut milk to blend it and add to the sauce.

Add chilies to the sauce (you can leave them whole or chop).

Bring back to a simmer and stir in the shrimp. Poach them stirring gently until they are opaque and just cooked (2-4 minutes only).

(garnishes, little red chili's and sprigs of dill).

- *Roasted curry powder:
- 2 Tbs whole coriander seeds
- 1 teas whole black peppercorns
- 1/4 tsp whole fenugreek seeds (I use powdered)
- 1 Tbs red paprika
- 1/4 to 1 teas cayenne pepper (I use an Indian red pepper)
- 1/2 tsp turmeric pepper.

Set skillet over moderate head and when hot pour in coriander seeds, peppercorns and fenugreek. Roast in the dry pan, stirring for about 1 min until an aroma is released.

Pour onto a paper towel and let cool. Grind spices in a coffee mill or use a mortar and pestle to get a powder. Add remaining ingredients.

Tropical Grilled Shrimp Cocktail

YIELD

SERVES 4-6

PREP TIME 15 MINUTES | **TOTAL TIME** 40 MINUTES

INGREDIENTS

- 1 lb. uncooked large shrimp, peeled and deveined
- 2 Tbs. lime juice
- 1/2 tsp. grated lime peel
- 1 clove garlic, finely chopped
- 1/3 cup mayonnaise
- 1 medium mango, peeled and diced (about 2 cups)
- 1/2 medium fresh papaya, peeled and diced (about 2 cups)
- 1/3 cup red onion, finely chopped
- 1 Tbs. chopped flat-leaf parsley

DIRECTIONS

Toss shrimp with 1 tablespoon of lime juice, lime peel, garlic and 1 tablespoon of mayonnaise. Marinate 15 minutes. Remove shrimp from marinade, discarding marinade. Grill or broil, turning once, until shrimp turn pink; set aside.

Meanwhile, in medium bowl, combine mango, papaya, red onion, remaining Mayonnaise, remaining 1 tablespoon of lime juice and parsley. To serve, spoon mango mixture into margarita glasses or glass dishes and evenly top with shrimp. Garnish, if desired, with lime wedges.

....

Island Barbequed Shrimp

YIELD

SERVES 4

PREP TIME 5 MINUTES | **TOTAL TIME** 20 MINUTES

INGREDIENTS

- 1 lb. shrimp, jumbo or large, cleaned, tails on.
- 2 Tbs olive oil
- 1 Tbs garlic, finely minced
- 1 Tbs rosemary, chopped fresh
- 1/2 tsp. thyme, chopped fresh
- 1/4 tsp. cayenne pepper, or to taste
- 1/4 tsp. salt
- 2 limes, halved

DIRECTIONS

Combine all except shrimp and limes. Marinate at room temperature for *1 hour. Heat a dry skillet over medium-high heat. When skillet is hot, lay the shrimp in pan. Cook shrimp 2-4 minutes per side. Brush with remaining marinade before turning. Serve with lime.

Coconut Shrimp

YIELD

SERVES 4-5

PREP TIME 5 MINUTES | **TOTAL TIME** 20 MINUTES

INGREDIENTS

- 1-1/2 lb. raw prawns (or shrimp)
- 2 cups thick coconut milk
- 1 Tbs. minced garlic
- 1 tsp. minced ginger root
- 1 tsp. salt
- 1/4 tsp. black pepper

DIRECTIONS

Wash shrimp but do not shell them. Place into a saucepan with coconut milk, garlic, ginger, salt and pepper. Bring to a boil, stirring. Reduce heat and simmer uncovered 15 minutes. Stir frequently.

Crab Stuffed Portobello Mushrooms

YIELD
SERVES 4
PREP TIME 5 MINUTES | **TOTAL TIME** 25 MINUTES

INGREDIENTS

- 6-12 oz. crab (1-2 cups, depending on how much meat you need)
- 10 oz. package frozen chopped spinach (I cooked my own fresh)
- 1 ½ lb. portobello mushrooms
- 1/4 cup chopped onions
- 2 cloves garlic, minced (I put in 2 teaspoons of already minced garlic)
- 1/2 teaspoon dried basil,
- 1/2 dried oregano,
- 1/4 teaspoon ground ginger
- 1/4 cup white wine
- 1 tablespoons fresh squeezed lemon juice

DIRECTIONS

Thaw spinach (or cook) then drain well by squeezing access liquid from it.

Remove stems from mushrooms (in case with extra large Portobello mushrooms, also, carve out some of the insides with a spoon). Set tops aside. Chop enough mushroom stems to make 2 cups. In a skillet, cook the chopped mushrooms stems, onion and garlic with the white wine and lemon juice until onion is tender but not browned.

Add the thawed spinach. Cook over low heat until most of the liquid is fully evaporated. (If still too much then set aside excess in extra bowl but leave some in skillet).

Now Stir the basil, oregano and the ginger into the spinach mixture until saturated.

Add the crab and stir until mixed (stirring too much will cause crab to separate and disappear into mixture).

Spoon the mixture into the mushrooms tops.

Place stuffed mushroom tops in the nonstick baking pan or casserole. Brush access liquid over sides and top of stuffed mushrooms. Bake in a 425 degree F oven for 10-15 minutes (20 minutes if extra large portobello) or until mushrooms are tender.

Coconut Lobster

YIELD

SERVES 4

PREP TIME 15 MINUTES | **TOTAL TIME** 30 MINUTES

YIELD

SERVES 4

TAKES up to 24 MINUTES

INGREDIENTS

- Meat of 4 medium-sized cooked lobsters, shelled and cut into chunks.
- 1/2 cup nut milk (optional)
- 1 cup coconut milk
- 1 small onion, finely chopped
- 2 scallions, finely chopped
- 2 springs thyme
- 2 tablespoons curry powder
- Salt and freshly ground white or black pepper to taste
- Dash cayenne pepper
- Fresh lime or lemon wedges

DIRECTIONS

Preheat oven to 400 F. Mix the nut milk and coconut milk together. Heat in a large saucepan over moderate heat. Add the onion, scallions, thyme, and curry powder. Stir and cook for about 5 min.

Add the lobster chunks, salt, pepper and cayenne. Cook slowly for 7-8 min. so that all flavors are well blended. Remove to a baking dish.

Bake for about 15 min. or until lobster is browned. Serve with lime or lemon wedges. Serve in the lobster shells.

Mussels in Hot Pepper Sauce

YIELD

SERVES 4

PREP TIME 5 MINUTES | **TOTAL TIME** 25 MINUTES

INGREDIENTS

- 2 quarts mussels
- 1-2 cups water
- 1 Tbs. olive oil
- 1 large garlic clove
- 1/2 cup chopped onion
- 6 oz. tomato paste
- 2 1/2 cups liquid from the mussels
- 1/2 tsp. oregano
- 1/4 tsp. (or to taste) crushed red pepper flakes, crushed

DIRECTIONS

Rinse mussels in colander several times with cold water. Place mussels in pan with 1-2 cups water; steam until open. Reserve the liquid, add enough water to make 2 1/2 cups liquid and set aside. Heat oil. Sauté the garlic and onion. Add the remaining ingredients and simmer 30 minutes. Put mussels, in their shells, in a shallow baking dish. Cover with sauce. Bake at 425F for 15 minutes. Serve on the half-shell. Note: It might be necessary to strain the reserved broth.

Steamed Chili Mussels in White wine and Garlic

Lisa's Recipe

YIELD

SERVES 4

PREP TIME 5 MINUTES | **TOTAL TIME** 30 MINUTES

INGREDIENTS

- 1 tsp extra-virgin olive oil.
- 4 Cloves garlic, finely chopped or pressed
- 1 Hand Full of Fresh Parsley finely cut.
- 1 Tbs of a quality chili powder*.
- 11/2 cups white wine, I use pinot grigio or Moscato
- 1 cup filtered water
- 1/2 tsp Salt
- 1/2 tsp Pepper
- 3 lbs. live mussels, rinsed.
- Small Leak chopped or other vegetable

DIRECTIONS

Add the above ingredients to an extra large pan with a lid. After rinsing the muscles add them to the pan and ONLY THEN place on a medium / low heat. Bring to the boil, this mixes and infuses the herbs and garlic and adds flavor to the mussels. Boil for approx. 20–25 minute max. (make sure that the mussels are opened and sample one from the center to your required taste). Always discard any unopened or broken mussels.

Serve from the pan and enjoy the sauce with a Grain free Paleo bread and garlic
*(Alternatively, you can use paprika for a delicious spicy taste.)

Steamed Mussels in Tomato Broth

YIELD
SERVES 4

PREP TIME 5 MINUTES | **TOTAL TIME** 30 MINUTES

INGREDIENTS

- 1 teaspoon extra-virgin olive oil
- 4 cloves garlic, finely chopped
- 6 ripe plum tomatoes, cored and coarsely chopped
- 1 cup dry white wine
- 3 pounds mussels, scrubbed and de bearded
- 2 teaspoons chopped fresh parsley

DIRECTIONS

Warm oil in a large pot with a tight-fitting lid over low heat. Add garlic and cook, stirring, until golden, about 3 minutes. Add tomatoes, increase
the heat to high and stir for 1 minute more. Pour in wine and bring to a boil.

Add mussels, cover and steam, occasionally giving the pan a vigorous shake, until all the mussels have opened, up to 20-25 minutes max. Discard any that do not open. Transfer the mussels to a serving bowl. Spoon the broth over the mussels and sprinkle with parsley.

Tip: To clean mussels, run under cold water inside a colander 1-2 minutes. I personally like my seafood to taste of the sea so don't over do this if you prefer that taste.
Or scrub them with a stiff brush under cold running water. Scrape off any barnacles using the shell of another mussel. Just before cooking, pull off the "beard" from each one.
Always discard any mussels with broken shells or any that do not close when tapped.

Poached Cod

YIELD

SERVES 2

PREP TIME 6 MINUTES | **TOTAL TIME** 24 MINUTES

INGREDIENTS

- 2 Pieces of Fresh Cod
- 2 Cloves Garlic
- 1 Tablespoon of Coconut oil
- 1 Med ripe tomato
- 2 table spoons of Fresh Parsley
- 1 Medium zucchini,
- 1 Cup of calamata olives
- Juice of half a lime (optional)
- Pinch salt and pepper.

DIRECTIONS

Preheat oven to 350F.

In an oven safe dish combine cod, sliced tomatoes, olive oil, and minced garlic, parsley, chopped zucchini, calamata olives, juice of half a lime (optional) salt and pepper. Poach until fish flakes easily when tested with a fork.

....

Macadamia-Crusted Salmon

YIELD

SERVES 4

PREP TIME 10 MINUTES | **TOTAL TIME** 34 MINUTES

INGREDIENTS

- 1 - 1 1/2 pounds salmon fillets, skin removed if possible
- 1 Cup raw macadamia nuts, chopped
- 1 Lemon

- 1 tsp. dried basil (or 1 T fresh)
- 1 tsp. dried parsley (or 1 T fresh)
- Sea salt and black pepper to taste
- 2 Teaspoon virgin olive oil
- Dijon mustard

DIRECTIONS

Heat oven to 400° F

Place salmon, skin side down if not removed, on a foil or parchment lined roasting pan

Mix together nuts, zest, herbs, salt and pepper in a small bowl. Add oil and combine.

Coat fish with a thin layer of mustard (or mayonnaise) and cover with nut mixture. Bake for 20 minutes.

....

Cajun Baked Catfish

YIELD

SERVES 2

PREP TIME 10 MINUTES | **TOTAL TIME** 30 MINUTES

INGREDIENTS

- 2 tablespoons almond meal
- 2 teaspoons Cajun seasoning or blackening seasoning
- 1/2 teaspoon dried thyme
- 1/2 teaspoon dried basil
- 1/4 teaspoon garlic powder
- 1/4 teaspoon lemon-pepper seasoning
- 2 catfish fillets (6 ounces each)
- 1/4 teaspoon paprika

DIRECTIONS

In a large re-sealable plastic bag, combine the almond meal, Cajun seasoning, thyme, basil, garlic powder and lemon-pepper. Add catfish and shake to coat.

Place on a baking sheet coated with cooking spray. Sprinkle with paprika. Bake at 400° for 20-25 minutes or until the fish flakes easily with a fork.

....

Salmon with Leeks

YIELD
SERVES 2

PREP TIME 10 MINUTES | **TOTAL TIME** 44 MINUTES

INGREDIENTS

- 2 salmon fillets
- 2 Julienne medium size leeks
- 1 Lime or Lemon
- 11/2 Tablespoon Coconut oil
- Crushed Fresh Ginger root
- Salt and pepper to taste.

DIRECTIONS

Julienne medium size leeks and wash thoroughly in strainer.
Preheat oven to 450°F.
Place the salmon fillets in an oven-safe dish and marinate in lime or lemon juice, olive oil, minced fresh ginger, salt and pepper.
Marinate covered in refrigerator at least 30 minutes.
Meanwhile, blanch the leeks in boiling water for 3 minutes and drain.
Toss leeks with olive oil, lime or lemon juice, salt and pepper.
Remove salmon to a plate and pour leeks and marinade into the oven-safe dish.
Place salmon on top of leeks skin side down.
Bake until cooked through, about 15-20 minutes or until fish flakes easily when tested with a fork.
Sprinkle with minced chives or parsley.
Decorate with lemon or lime slices if desired.

Rainbow Trout

Whole rainbow trout, no head or tail and filleted, but one whole piece.
Place some extra virgin olive oil inside the fish.

YIELD

SERVES 2

PREP TIME 7 MINUTES | **TOTAL TIME** 22 MINUTES

INGREDIENTS

- Pepper
- Lemon slices
- Tomato slices
- Rosemary
- Thyme

DIRECTIONS

Close the trout, place in parchment paper tightly sealed and baked at 350F for about 15 minutes.

Tuna Amandine

YIELD

SERVES 6

PREP TIME 14 MINUTES | **TOTAL TIME** 44 MINUTES

INGREDIENTS

- 1 bunch asparagus spears, cooked just until tender
- 1 9-ounce can tuna packed in water, drained and flaked
- 1/2 cup rendered fat
- 1/2 cup blanched almonds, chopped
- 5 tablespoons arrowroot
- 1 teaspoon salt
- 1/4 teaspoon pepper
- 1/8 teaspoon nutmeg

- 3 cups coconut milk or almond milk
- 2 tablespoons dry sherry
- 1 teaspoon Paprika

DIRECTIONS

Preheat oven to 350 degrees F. grease a 1-1/2 quart baking dish thoroughly.

Arrange asparagus spears on the bottom of prepared dish. Cover with tuna.

Lightly brown almonds in fat. Blend in arrowroot, salt, pepper, and nutmeg. Add milk, stirring constantly. Cook until smooth and thick. Stir in sherry.
Pour sauce over tuna. Sprinkle with paprika. Bake 30 minutes.
Makes about 6 servings

Mackerel Pizzaiola

YIELD

SERVES 4
PREP TIME 20 MINUTES | **TOTAL TIME** 40 MINUTES

INGREDIENTS

- 2 whole mackerel, 1 1/2 to 2 pounds each
- 3 garlic cloves, chopped
- 1 Tbs. chopped fresh parsley
- Salt and pepper to taste
- 2 tsp. chopped fresh oregano or 1/2 tsp. dried
- 2 Tbs. chopped fresh basil or 1/2 tsp. dried
- 1 (14 oz.) can Italian peeled tomatoes, drained and chopped

DIRECTIONS

Preheat oven to 350F. Slash mackerel diagonally, 3 times on each side, to 1 inch deep. Place fish in an oiled 13" x 9" baking dish. Cover fish with tomatoes, garlic, basil, parsley and pepper. Bake 35 minutes, or until fish flakes when tested with a fork. Serve with pan sauce.

Salmon with Spinach Green Sauce

YIELD

SERVES 4

PREP TIME 20 MINUTES | **TOTAL TIME** 40 MINUTES

INGREDIENTS

- 2 salmon Fillets
- 11/2 handful spinach or watercress
- 2/3 sprigs fresh parsley
- 2 shallots
- 1 Tbs lemon juice
- salt and pepper.

DIRECTIONS

Brush salmon fillet with olive oil and grill.
Garnish with fresh dill and lemon juice.
Sauce: In your food processor mix
spinach or watercress, fresh parsley, shallots, lemon juice, salt and pepper. Chill and serve as dip to accompany fish.

Poached Swordfish with Lemon Parsley Sauce

YIELD

SERVES 2

PREP TIME 12 MINUTES | **TOTAL TIME** 30* MINUTES

INGREDIENTS

- 2 fresh sword fish fillets min 150 grams each

In a small bowl, combine
- dash coconut oil / extra virgin olive
- 1 teaspoon lemon juice

- 11/2 tablespoon minced flat leaf parsley
- ½ teaspoon salt and freshly ground black pepper.

DIRECTIONS

Set aside for no more than 30 minutes* or the lemon juice will yellow the parsley. Bring 3-4 cups of water to a boil in a saucepan large enough to fit the fish pieces comfortably. Holding the fish with a slotted spoon lower gently into the pan and bring the water back to a boil.

Reduce the heat to very low and poach the fish for 3-4 minutes until barely cooked through. Lift the fish from the water, drain thoroughly and arrange each fillet on a warm plate. Spoon the sauce over the fish and serve immediately.

Grilled Sword Fish with Orange Salad

YIELD

SERVES 4

PREP TIME 12 MINUTES | **TOTAL TIME** 24 MINUTES

INGREDIENTS

- 2 Tbs. finely chopped red onion pinch of crushed red pepper
- 2 Tbs. Coconut Oil / extra-virgin olive oil
- 2 tsp. fresh lemon juice
- 1/2 tsp. pepper
- 3 large navel oranges
- 8 oil-cured black olives, pitted and coarsely chopped
- 1/2 cup fresh mint leaves, chopped (2 Tbs.)
- 4 (1/2 inch thick) swordfish steaks, about 6 oz. each

DIRECTIONS

With a sharp knife, peel oranges, making sure to remove the white pith.

Holding oranges over a medium bowl, remove sections by cutting along membranes with a small knife, letting sections fall into bowl. Stir in the olives, mint, onion, crushed pepper, 1 Tbs. of the oil and the lemon juice.

Refrigerate. Heat grill to HIGH and brush with about 1/2 of the oil. Brush swordfish with the other half, and sprinkle with pepper. Grill fish 2-3 minutes on each side, or just until cooked thru. Transfer fish to serving plates, top with the orange, olive, mint salad and serve.

....

Fish Burgers

Put them in the fridge for a while before cooking them, makes a refreshing change from regular beef burgers

YIELD

SERVES 8-10

PREP TIME 10 MINUTES | **TOTAL TIME** 22 MINUTES

INGREDIENTS

- 240g drained canned tuna
- 1/2 cup finely chopped onion
- 1/4 cup finely chopped red capsicum Pepper
- 1 egg, lightly beaten
- 1/4 cup finely chopped celery
- 1 tsp. finely chopped fresh dill
- 3 tsp. lemon juice
- 1 Tbs coconut oil.

DIRECTIONS

Combine all ingredients in a bowl. Form mixture into four equal patties.
Heat oil on barbecue hot plate until hot. Barbecue tuna patties 8-10 minutes, turning once.

Curried Scallops in Coconut Milk

YIELD

SERVES 2-4

PREP TIME 10 MINUTES | **TOTAL TIME** 20 MINUTES

INGREDIENTS

- Oil for sautéing
- 1 TB Ginger root, finely chopped
- 2 cloves Garlic, finely chopped
- 1/2 tsp. Crushed red pepper or chili pepper
- 1 tsp. Curry powder
- 1 cup Scallops, marinated in juice of 2 limes
- Sea salt to taste
- 1 cup Vegetable broth or if preferred water
- 1/2 cup Coconut milk
- Sliced green onions for garnish

DIRECTIONS

1. Sauté the ginger and garlic in oil for one minute.
2. Add the spices and sauté for another minute.
3. Add the scallops and sea salt and sauté for 1 minute.
4. Add coconut milk, broth and slowly bring to boil. Turn down heat and simmer for a few minutes until scallops are cooked.
5. Garnish each dish with slivered green onions.

Other seafood such as shrimp or calamari (squid) can easily be substituted for scallops. Experiment with your favorite spices such as cayenne, cumin or turmeric to create your very own recipe.

Avocado and Scallop Ceviche

YIELD
SERVES 2-4
PREP TIME 20 MINUTES | **TOTAL TIME** 48 MINUTES *

INGREDIENTS

- 1/2 c Lime juice
- 3 Tsp Olive oil
- 24 Green peppercorns; crushed
- Salt and pepper, to taste
- 3/4 lb. Bay scallops, chopped
- 1 large Avocado; peeled
- 2 Tbs Chives, chopped
- 40 small Mushrooms
- 1/4 cup Coconut oil / Olive oil
- 2 Tbs Lemon juice
- 1 med Garlic clove

DIRECTIONS

Combine lime-juice, oil, peppercorns, salt and pepper together in a glass or ceramic bowl. Stir in the scallops, cover and refrigerate for at least 4 hours while they marinate.* They should become opaque in this time.

Mash the avocado until almost smooth, then add it along with the chives or scallions to the marinating scallops (do not drain them) and mix well. Set aside for at least 1/2 hour, refrigerated.

About half an hour before serving the scallops, remove the stems from the mushrooms and wipe them to remove any dirt combine the vegetable oil, lemon juice, garlic, salt and pepper in a small bowl, and brush the insides of the mushrooms liberally with the mixture. Just before serving, drain the caps and fill with the scallop mixture. Garnish with additional chives, if desired.

Scallops in Coconut-Basil Sauce

YIELD

SERVES 4-6

PREP TIME 14 MINUTES | **TOTAL TIME** 22 MINUTES

INGREDIENTS

- 2 (14-ounce) cans unsweetened coconut milk
- 1 tablespoon grated fresh ginger
- 1/4 cup fresh lime juice
- 1/4 teaspoon ground red pepper
- 2 pounds sea scallops
- 1 tablespoon pure fish sauce, e.g. Red Boat Fish Sauce
- 2 tablespoons chopped fresh basil

DIRECTIONS

Combine first 4 ingredients in a 12-inch, straight-sided skillet; bring to a boil. Reduce heat to medium-low or until mixture simmers. Add scallops; cover and poach at a light simmer, adjusting heat as necessary, for 8 minutes or until scallops turn opaque.

Using a slotted spoon, remove scallops from skillet; place in a shallow dish or individual serving bowls. Cover with foil. Boil coconut-milk mixture over high heat, uncovered, for 10 to 15 minutes or until reduced to 1 1/2 cups. Stir in fish sauce and basil; spoon over scallops.

CHAPTER 16

PALEO SALAD RECIPES
Fresh Mushroom Salad

YIELD
SERVES 3-4
PREP TIME 10 MINUTES | TOTAL TIME 18 MINUTES

INGREDIENTS

- 2/3 cup olive oil
- 1/3 cup fresh lemon juice
- 1 tsp. dried thyme
- Salt and pepper to taste
- 1 pound fresh mushrooms, thinly sliced
- 1/4 cup minced parsley
- ½ Lettuce

DIRECTIONS

Combine all ingredients except the mushrooms, parsley and lettuce, and mix well. Add the mushrooms and toss with 2 forks. Cover and let stand at room temperature.

At serving time, drain and sprinkle with the parsley. Pile in a serving dish lined with lettuce.

....

Sunny Apple Salad

YIELD
SERVES 4
PREP TIME 12 MINUTES | TOTAL TIME 16 MINUTES

INGREDIENTS

- 2 medium red apples, diced
- 1 medium green apple, diced
- 1 medium carrot, grated
- 1 can (8 oz.) crushed pineapple, drained
- 3 Tablespoons orange juice concentrate

DIRECTIONS

In a bowl, combine all ingredients; mix well. Cover and refrigerate until serving.

Avocado Salad

YIELD
SERVES 6
PREP TIME 8MINUTES | TOTAL TIME 38 MINUTES

INGREDIENTS

- 2 avocados, halved, pitted, peeled and diced
- 1 medium tomato, diced
- 3/4 cup coarsely chopped fresh cilantro
- 1/2 cup finely diced onion
- 2 teaspoons finely chopped jalapeño
- 1-1/2 tablespoons fresh lime juice
- 1/2 teaspoon of salt

DIRECTIONS

In a medium bowl, combine avocados, tomato, cilantro, onion and jalapeño.
Add lime juice and salt; mix well. Cover and chill for at least 30 minutes.
Ideas:
Serve this flavorful salad on a bed of mixed greens or in a large lettuce cup for a light lunch. It is also excellent with grilled meats.

Cranberry Apple Salad

YIELD

SERVES 6-8

PREP TIME 10 MINUTES | TOTAL TIME 22 MINUTES

INGREDIENTS

- 2 Tablespoons agar-agar flakes or gelatin
- 2 cups fresh apple juice
- 1 cup cranberries
- 2/3 cup diced pineapple
- 2/3 cup grapefruit sections, diced
- 1 cup celery, chopped
- 2 Tablespoons raw honey

DIRECTIONS

Soften agar or gelatin in a half cup of apple juice. Heat remaining juice and add to gelatin. Mash cranberries and add to gelatin with other fruits, celery and honey. Pour into 1-1/2 quart mold. Chill until firm. Unmold and serve.

....

Strawberry Fields Salad

YIELD

SERVES 4

PREP TIME 10 MINUTES | TOTAL TIME 14 MINUTES

INGREDIENTS

- 1 (11-ounce) can mandarin oranges, drained
- 1 pint fresh strawberries, stemmed and quartered
- 1 small red onion, thinly sliced
- 1/2 cup coarsely chopped pecans, toasted
- 1 avocado, sliced

- 1 package romaine lettuce

A cinnamon dressing is recommended.

....

Tomato Salad Curry

YIELD

SERVES 4

PREP TIME 10 MINUTES | TOTAL TIME 14 MINUTES*

INGREDIENTS

- 6 large ripe tomatoes, peeled, seeded and chopped
- 1 small white onion, grated
- 1/4 tsp. coarsely ground pepper
- 1/2 cup mayonnaise
- 2 Tbs. minced fresh parsley
- 1 tsp. curry powder

DIRECTIONS

Combine tomatoes, onion and pepper; cover and chill for 3 hours.* To serve, spoon tomato mixture into small bowls and top each with a spoonful of mayonnaise mixture.

....

Apple Coleslaw

YIELD

SERVES 4

PREP TIME 10 MINUTES | TOTAL TIME 14 MINUTES

INGREDIENTS

- 2 cups packaged coleslaw mix (bag of chopped cabbage, in produce section)
- 1 unpeeled tart apple, chopped

- 1/2 cup chopped celery
- 1/2 cup chopped green pepper
- 1/4 cup olive oil
- 2 tablespoons lemon juice
- 2 tablespoons raw honey
- 1 teaspoon celery seed

DIRECTIONS

In a bowl, combine the coleslaw mix, apple, celery and green pepper. In a small bowl, whisk remaining ingredients. Pour over coleslaw and toss to coat. Makes approx. 4-6 servings.

SALADS AND SIDES

Crab and Cucumber Salad

YIELD

SERVES 4

PREP TIME 8 MINUTES | TOTAL TIME 18 MINUTES

INGREDIENTS

- 4 oz. crab classic flake style
- 1 large cucumber, peeled, seeded and sliced
- 1 medium onion, diced
- 1 yellow pepper, diced
- 1 Tbs. lemon or lime juice
- salt and pepper to taste

DIRECTIONS

Place crab classic in a bowl and break flakes into smaller pieces. Add cucumber, onion and pepper and mix. Add 1 tablespoon of lemon juice, salt and pepper to taste and toss.

Shrimp Cocktail

YIELD

SERVES 4

PREP TIME 8 MINUTES | **TOTAL TIME** 18 MINUTES

INGREDIENTS

- 1 pound shrimp
- 6 Tbs. chili sauce
- 2 Tbs. lemon juice
- 1/2 Tbs. horseradish
- 1/4 teaspoon grated onion
- 1/3 cup finely chopped celery
- Crisp salad greens (2 cups leaves)
- lemon wedges

DIRECTIONS

Cook and clean shrimp, cover and chill. Combine chili sauce, lemon juice, horseradish, and onion to make cocktail sauce. Stir. Mix chilled shrimp with celery. Line cocktail cups with salad greens. Spoon in shrimp mixture. Spoon on some sauce. Garnish with lemon wedges.

The Manhattan Avocado Cocktail

YIELD

SERVES 4

PREP TIME 10 MINUTES | **TOTAL TIME** 22 MINUTES

INGREDIENTS

- 1/4 cup extra-virgin olive oil
- 1 garlic clove, mashed
- 1/2 teaspoon cumin
- 2 tablespoons fresh lime juice
- 3/4 teaspoon salt

- 1 pound cooked jumbo shrimp
- 2 teaspoons minced red Thai or jalapeno chili pepper
- 2 avocados, halved, pitted, peeled and sliced
- 3 ounces mesculin greens (2 cups, slightly packed)
- 1/2 cup seeded and diced tomato for garnish

DIRECTIONS

In a microwave-proof cup, microwave the oil, garlic and cumin seeds, on high, 30 seconds to 1 minute, just until hot. Let stand 10 minutes. Remove the garlic with a fork, whisk in the lime juice and salt. In a medium bowl, toss shrimp with 1 tablespoon of the dressing and the chili pepper. Cover
and refrigerate. Place avocado slices in a 9" glass pie plate. Drizzle with
2 tablespoons of the dressing, (whisking first with fork to blend). Shake dish to coat avocado. Press plastic wrap lightly over surface of avocado and seal around edge of plate. Refrigerate up to 4 hours. Reserve remaining dressing.

To serve: Toss greens with 1 tablespoon of remaining dressing. Divide greens among 4 martini glasses, mounding in center. Arrange shrimp and dot with tomato. Decoratively stand avocado slices in glass, using the greens and shrimp to rest on.

For scallops: In a large non-stick skillet, heat 1-teaspoon olive oil over medium-high heat. Sprinkle scallops with 1-2 minutes per side, until lightly browned. Cool. Proceed with recipe, adding the dressing.

Cold Shrimp Stuffed Avocados

YIELD

SERVES 6

PREP TIME 14 MINUTES | **TOTAL TIME** 24 MINUTES

YIELD

SERVES 6

TAKES up to 24 MINUTES

INGREDIENTS

- 3 large avocados
- juice of 1 lemon
- 1 pound cooked shelled shrimp (reserve 6 whole shrimp), coarsely chopped
- 1 hot chili pepper, peeled if fresh, seeded, washed and chopped fine
- 1 hard-cooked egg, chopped
- 2 dozen pitted green or black olives, chopped
- Paleo mayonnaise
- Pinch pepper
- 3 Tbs. minced fresh coriander leaves or parsley

DIRECTIONS

Cut avocados in half lengthwise, pit, and scoop out the flesh. Put the flesh into a bowl, now sprinkle the shells with a little lemon juice to prevent darkening. Mash the avocado flesh with a fork. Add the shrimp, hot pepper, egg and olives and mix well. Add enough mayonnaise, beginning with 1/3 cup, to bind the ingredients together. Pepper to taste. Stuff the avocado shells with this mixture. Top each with one of the reserved shrimp and sprinkle with coriander. 6 servings.

Paleo Tuna Salad

YIELD

SERVES 2-4
PREP TIME 10 MINUTES | **TOTAL TIME** 22 MINUTES

INGREDIENTS

- 1 medium onion
- 2 stalks celery
- nutmeg
- Pinch salt and pepper
- 1 Tbs olive oil
- 2 cans plain tuna
- 1/3 cup finely chopped walnuts
- 1/3-3/4 cup paleo made mayonnaise (depending on how creamy you like it)

DIRECTIONS

Chop up the onion and celery, then pan fry it in the olive oil, with some nutmeg, salt, and pepper. Put it in the refrigerator to cool, if you prefer cold salad. Drain the tuna, and mix all of the ingredients together.

Makes 2 large servings or 4 small servings. It's yummy stuff and makes for a great weekend lunch.

Chicken Waldorf Salad

YIELD
SERVES 4
PREP TIME 15 MINUTES | **TOTAL TIME** 16 MINUTES*

INGREDIENTS

- 2 cups of cooked diced chicken*
- 1 large tart apple, cored and diced
- 1 cup chopped celery
- 1 cup grapes, halved and seeded [optional]
- 1/2 cup chopped walnuts [or pecan meat]
- 1/4 cup homemade mayonnaise [more if the next two are omitted]
- 2 tsp. lime juice [optional]
- 2 tsp. honey [optional]
- Pinch pepper

DIRECTIONS

In a medium size bowl, combine cooked chicken, apple, celery and walnuts. In a small bowl, combine mayonnaise, lime juice and honey; stir to blend well. Season to taste with pepper. Spoon dressing over chicken salad, and toss to coat.

CHAPTER 17

SAUCES AND DIPS

Almond Hummus

YIELD

SERVES 2-4

PREP TIME 10 MINUTES | **TOTAL TIME** 18 MINUTES*

INGREDIENTS

- 2 cups almonds, soaked for 12 hours, then rinsed*
- 2/3 cup raw organic tahini
- 1/2 cup water
- 2 cloves garlic
- Juice of 2 small lemons
- 1/2 teaspoon sea salt
- 1/4 cup chopped fresh parsley or cilantro

DIRECTIONS

Combine all ingredients in a food processor and puree. This almond hummus serves as a nice dip for raw veggies.

···

Macadamia Nut Hummus

YIELD

SERVES 2-4

PREP TIME 5 MINUTES | TOTAL TIME 15 MINUTES

INGREDIENTS

- 1 1/2 cups macadamia nuts, coarsely chopped
- 2 Tbs. lemon juice
- 2 Tbs. olive oil

- 1 clove garlic / ½ tsp. salt

DIRECTIONS

Place the nuts, lemon juice, olive oil and garlic in a food processor or high-performance blender and process to breakup the nuts somewhat. Add the sea salt.

Add about 1/2 cup water and process again until smooth. Add more water if the mixture is too thick. Taste for seasoning and add more lemon juice or sea salt if needed.

Place in the refrigerator to chill for about 30 minutes before enjoying.

··

Walnut Hummus

YIELD

SERVES 2-4

PREP TIME 10 MINUTES | TOTAL TIME 20 MINUTES

(Best 24hrs later)*

INGREDIENTS

- 1 1/2 cups raw walnut pieces or halves
- 2 tablespoons tahini
- 2 tablespoons lemon juice
- 1 tablespoon olive oil
- 1 garlic clove, chopped
- 1/2 teaspoon hot paprika
- 1/2 teaspoon salt
- black pepper

DIRECTIONS

In a food processor, process walnuts, tahini, lemon juice, olive oil, garlic, paprika and salt until smooth, about 30 seconds. Scrape down sides of the bowl as necessary.

Season to taste with salt and pepper. Pulse to blend. Transfer to a serving bowl. Serve immediately, or cover and refrigerate up to 1 day*.

Avocado Salsa

YIELD

SERVES 2-4

PREP TIME 5 MINUTES | TOTAL TIME 14 MINUTES

INGREDIENTS

- 1 large avocado, finely diced
- 1/2 small red onion, finely diced
- 2 tablespoons chopped coriander leaves
- Squeeze lime juice

DIRECTIONS

Combine all ingredients in a bowl, season to taste with lime juice, salt and black pepper. Toss gently to combine.

....

Guacamole

YIELD

SERVES 2-4

PREP TIME 5 MINUTES | TOTAL TIME 14 MINUTES

INGREDIENTS

- 4 large ripe avocados, flesh
- 1/2 large red onion, roughly chopped
- 5 garlic cloves, crushed
- 1 jalapeño, seeds removed, roughly chopped
- 1/2 bunch cilantro leaves
- 2 tablespoons olive oil
- 2 limes, juiced
- 1/2 tablespoon kosher salt

DIRECTIONS

Combine avocado, red onion, garlic, jalapeño, and cilantro in a food processor and pulse to mix. While the processor is running, add olive oil, lime juice and salt. Remove guacamole from food processor and serve. Makes 4 cups.

....

Guacamole-Topped Bacon Bites

YIELD
SERVES 2-4
PREP TIME 5 MINUTES | **TOTAL TIME** 20 MINUTES

INGREDIENTS

- 1 lb. of bacon strips
- guacamole

DIRECTIONS

Preheat oven to 375 degrees. Cut bacon strips into thirds and arrange them on a baking sheet lined with parchment paper.

Bake the bacon for 10 to 15 minutes or until very crispy. Remove and place on paper towels to blot grease.

Put a spoonful of guacamole on a piece of bacon, and top with another piece of bacon. Repeat until all bacon has been done.

....

Cauliflower Hummus

YIELD
SERVES 2
PREP TIME 10 MINUTES | **TOTAL TIME** 20 MINUTES

INGREDIENTS

- 1/5 head of cauliflower
- 2 Tbs sesame tahini
- 1/2 clove of garlic

- 1/8 cup water
- Dash of lemon juice
- 1 Tbs olive oil
- Tomato, diced (optional)
- Ground cumin (optional)

DIRECTIONS

Boil or steam cauliflower until cooked. Put cauliflower into food processor with sesame tahini and garlic. Add water. Start to process. Add lemon juice and a tablespoon of olive oil and process until it gets creamy. Add more oil if you want to improve the texture.

Zucchini Spread

YIELD

SERVES 4-6

PREP TIME 10 MINUTES | **TOTAL TIME** 22 MINUTES

INGREDIENTS

- 3 1/2 cups zucchini (unpeeled shredded equiv. to 1 pound)
- 1/4 cup fresh parsley (finely snipped)
- 2 Tbs lemon juice
- 1 Tbs. olive oil
- 1 garlic clove (minced)
- 1/4 tsp. salt
- Pinch pepper
- 2 Tbs finely chopped pecans [or walnuts]

DIRECTIONS

Squeeze the zucchini to remove excess water.
In a food processor or blender, process the zucchini and all other ingredients except the nuts until smooth, scraping the sides as needed.
Spoon the mixture into a serving bowl. Fold in the nuts. Cover and refrigerate before serving.

Roasted-Red-Pepper Dip

YIELD
SERVES 2-4
PREP TIME 10 MINUTES | **TOTAL TIME** 22 MINUTES

INGREDIENTS

- 6 large red bell peppers
- 1 cup golden raisins, coarsely chopped (6 ounces)
- 1/4 cup plus 2 tablespoons extra-virgin olive oil
- 3 tablespoons salt-packed capers, rinsed well
- 1 1/2 teaspoons coarsely chopped fresh oregano

DIRECTIONS

Roast peppers over a gas flame or under the broiler, turning occasionally, until charred all over, about 10 minutes. Transfer to a heatproof bowl, and cover with plastic wrap. Let stand until cool enough to handle. Peel and seed peppers. Pulse peppers in a food processor until coarsely chopped. Add raisins, oil, capers, and oregano. Pulse to combine.

CHAPTER 18

PALEO SWEETS & DESSERTS

Pastry (for 9" double-crust pie)

YIELD
SERVES 4-6
PREP TIME 15 MINUTES | **TOTAL TIME** 35 MINUTES

INGREDIENTS

- 2 1/2 cups almond flour
- 2/3 cup shortening, e.g. lard or coconut oil
- 1/4 teaspoon salt
- 1/3 cup water

DIRECTIONS

Combine flour and salt in a mixing bowl. Cut shortening into flour with a pastry blender or two knives. Do not over mix; these are sufficiently blended when particles are the size of peas. Add water gradually, sprinkling a little at a time over the mixture. Use only enough water to hold the pastry together when it is pressed between the fingers. It should NOT feel wet.

Roll dough into a round ball, handling as little as possible. Roll out on a lightly floured board into a circle 1/8 in thick and one inch larger than the diameter of the top of the pie pan.

Trim to the edge of the pie pan. Prick with a fork. Bake at 450F for 12 - 15 minutes or until a golden brown.

Chocolate & Banana Mousse

YIELD

SERVES 1-2

PREP TIME 8 MINUTES | **TOTAL TIME** 14 MINUTES*

INGREDIENTS

- 1 1/2 C & 2 Tbs of Almond or Coconut Milk
- 2 C of raw cashews (soaked over night)*
- ¼ C of raw honey
- 6 Tbs of Cocoa Powder
- 1 Ripe Banana
- 1/4 tsp. nutmeg
- 1 tsp. Cinnamon
- 1 tsp. Mint or orange Flavouring (Alternative Option)**
- 1 Pinch Sea Salt

DIRECTIONS

Combine all the above ingredients in your blender and blend until smooth.
(Add the cocoa powder first and then pour the remainder of the ingredients on top this makes for easier blending).
Refrigerate the Mousse for about an hour to properly set.
Now Spoon serve into serving bowls, you can top with Sliced banana or other fruit as you desire.** Enjoy!

Fresh Strawberry Pie

YIELD

SERVES 4-6

PREP TIME 10 MINUTES | **TOTAL TIME** 60 MINUTES

INGREDIENTS

Pie Shell:
- 1 cup raw almonds
- 1 cup soft, pitted dates
- 1/2 tsp. vanilla

DIRECTIONS

Grind the nuts in a food processor until finely chopped, add the dates and vanilla, and blend well. Press thinly into a pie plate (from center to the outside rim) to form the shell.

Binder:
- 7 or 8 Large ripe strawberries
- 5 soft dates, pitted
- 2 bananas, fairly ripe
- 1 Tbs. fresh lemon juice

DIRECTIONS

Blend all ingredients in food processor or blender until well mixed.

Fruit Filling:

Cut 2 pints of fresh strawberries into quarters, fold into binder and fill shell. Decorate with approximately 1/2 pint of quartered strawberries.
Cover with plastic wrap and store in refrigerator. Chill thoroughly before serving.

Summer Frozen Fruit Bars

YIELD

SERVES 4-6

PREP TIME 10 MINUTES | **TOTAL TIME** 60 MINUTES

INGREDIENTS

- 2 cups cut-up summer fruit (strawberries, peaches, watermelon, etc.)
- 1/2 tablespoon raw honey
- 1 teaspoon fresh lemon juice

DIRECTIONS

Place the fruit in a blender. Cover and blend until smooth.
Add 1-2 tablespoons water, if necessary. Add honey and lemon juice. Cover and blend until well mixed.
Pour into 4 oz. ice-pop molds or paper cups. Insert sticks. Freeze until solid.

....

Apple Ice Kreme

YIELD

SERVES 4-6

PREP TIME 10 MINUTES | **TOTAL TIME** 30 MINUTES

INGREDIENTS

This light and refreshing dessert takes a simple apple and makes you feel like you are eating something positively sinful.

- 2 cups applesauce (made by putting several peeled and cored apples through the Champion Juicer with blank)
- 2 cups apple juice
- 2 Tablespoons pure maple syrup (or less if sweet apples)
- 2 Teaspoons lemon juice

DIRECTIONS

Puree in blender or food processor. Place in shallow dish and freeze. Serve by scraping into curls with a soup spoon or ice cream scoop.

Variation: Add a scoop or two of Apple Ice Kreme to chilled Sparkling apple cider or apple juice for a special drink.

Note: You can also try this with peaches, strawberries, raspberries, blueberries, kiwi, oranges, tangerines, etc.

....

Avocado Pear Pops

YIELD

SERVES 6 PEOPLE

PREP TIME 5 MINUTES | **TOTAL TIME** 60 MINUTES

INGREDIENTS

- 2 avocado
- 2 pear (Peeled)

DIRECTIONS

Puree's the above then filled the molds half way, insert sticks, and freeze. Soak in hot water for a few seconds to remove from the mold.

Raw Banana Ice Cream

INGREDIENTS

The first time you make this you should eat it plain in order to appreciate the flavor. The times after that (and trust me, there will be many) you can dress it up with sauces and toppings.

This recipe makes one serving of ice cream - if you're making a larger batch of this ice cream for multiple people, just add one banana for each person*.

- 1 ripe banana
- 1 Tbs. flavoring
- Vanilla bean, chopped mint.
- 1/4 cup filling
- Strawberries, cherries, almonds, hazelnuts, walnuts, pecans, sliced
- bananas, coconut.
- 2 Tbs. sauce
- Strawberry sauce, almond butter and other nut butters.

DIRECTIONS

Slice banana into chunks, and place in a container. I actually do this every time I have ripe bananas lying around, so I always have a supply of frozen bananas ready in the freezer! The banana will take about 6-8 hours to freeze, so it's a good idea to do this step the night before.

Place banana chunks in food processor, and blend for about 5 minutes or until light and creamy in texture.

Eat ASAP, or place in the freezer for later. Keep in mind that it's preservative free, so it will tend to melt faster than regular ice creams and should be enjoyed immediately!

Fresh Fruit Frozen Dessert

YIELD

SERVES 1 PER BANANA

PREP TIME 5 MINUTES | **TOTAL TIME** 15 MINUTES

INGREDIENTS

- 1 frozen banana (To freeze, place unpeeled ripe banana in an air-tight
- freezer bag in the freezer)
- 1-2 tablespoons of chopped fruit of your choice.
- 1/2 tablespoon of chopped nuts (optional)

DIRECTIONS

Remove banana from the freezer and thaw for 1/2 hour. Peel and mash partially thawed banana with a fork. Add chopped fruit and nuts and stir.
Serve immediately. 1 serving (If you use more bananas, you can use a blender.)

....

Coconut Sorbet

YIELD

SERVES 1

PRE TIME 5 MINUTES | **TOTAL TIME** 15 MINUTES

INGREDIENTS

- 8 ounces coconut milk
- 16 ounces water
- 1/4 cup toasted coconut

DIRECTIONS

Combine the coconut milk and water and chill for several hours in the refrigerator.
Freeze the mixture in an ice cream freezer according to the manufacturer's instructions. Add the toasted coconut to the frozen coconut sorbet by stirring in using a spoon. Keep frozen until ready to serve.

Apple Crumble

YIELD

SERVES UP TO 6 PEOPLE

PREP TIME 15 MINUTES | **COOKING TIME** 30-40 MINUTES

INGREDIENTS

- 3-4 large granny smiths apples
- ½ juice of lemon
- 1 cup of almond meal / almond Flour
- ¼ cup of chopped macadamia or walnuts
- ¼ cup coconut oil / butter
- 1 tablespoon of raw organic honey
- ¼ teaspoon of cinnamon
- 2 pinches of sea salt

DIRECTIONS

Preheat oven at 375 f

Cut the apples in to slices or chucks as you prefer for consistency Squeeze the juice of the lemon over the apples.

In a large mixing bowl mix the almond meal / flour, macadamia nuts, melted butter, remaining lemon juice, raw honey, cinnamon and salt.

Spread the nut topping over the apples and bake until they are cooked / bubbly and the topping is golden brown about 30-40 minutes.

This recipes is one of my favorites, so I saved the best until last, I hope you like it.

Conclusion

Well that's the end of my Paleo Cookbook; I sincerely hope I gave you a valid account of our healthy ancient diet. I hope your well on your way to enjoying this evolutionary amazing food through the delicious recipes. If you have any questions about Paleo, or any of my books please email me directly, (See Below).

Also tell me how I can do better and make your reading more enjoyable, in my attempt to give you an exciting and thought provoking reading experience. I work to the continual improvement model from my many years in business (EFQM – European Foundation for Quality Management.

As you have gathered, I'm passionate about food and healthy eating I follow the Paleo diet EVERYDAY I am committed to eating the right foods that prevent so many of the diseases and ailments affecting us all This is my attempt to make us feel truly alive, every single day.

My appeal, if you really enjoyed my book please take a moment to leave me an honest review at the bottom of the amazon book description page. Reviews really do mean a lot.

Thank you each and every reader

With Love, to you, your health and happiness

Oliver

olivermichaels.author@hotmail.com

REFERENCE
RESOURCE INFORMATION.

[1] www.heart.org

[2]http://www.surgeongeneral.gov/library/calls/obesity/fact_consequences.html

[3]http://onlinelibrary.wiley.com/doi/10.1038/oby.2001.125/full

[4] http://www.posturecentre.ie/the-prevalence-of-childhood-obesity-in-adolescents/

[5] http://www.cdc.gov/HeartDisease/

[6] http://news.discovery.com/history/archaeology/human-ancestor-fire-120402.htm

[7] American Journal of Clinical Nutrition.

[8] Nutrition & Metabolism Society,

[9] Consumer report 2006 / 2010

http://www.consumerreports.org/cro/magazine-archive/2010/january/food/chicken-safety/overview/chicken-safety-ov.htm

[10 http://ajcn.nutrition.org/content/47/2/270.full.pdf

[11] http://www.ncbi.nlm.nih.gov/pubmed/2998440

[12] http://www.ncbi.nlm.nih.gov/pubmed/4111248

WORKS CITED AND CREDITED TO;-

https://www.ediets.com/celebrity-news/ediets-blog/2013/12/02/the-paleo-diet-a-weight-loss-hit-or-myth/
http://thehappyhealthfreak.com/2013/10/30/november-paleo-challenge-join-e/https://play.google.com/store/apps/details?id=com.paleodiet.ijavapp
http://answers.yahoo.com/question/index?qid=20120129001419AA9xUG1
http://www.prijatelji-ivotinja.hr/index.en.php?id=1165http://missearthsa.co.za/blog/?p=10928http://www.integratednaturalmedicine.com/6-benefits-eating-paleo/   http://paleogrubs.com/paleo-benefits   https://es-la.facebook.com/Manuelorsicoach http://www.telegraph.co.uk/health/healthnews/10428819/GPs-should-help-lead-obesity-fight-says-Jamie-Oliver.html
http://www.thepaleosecret.com/2012/11/05/the-paleo-secrets-top-10-keys-to-optimizing-digestion/

MEDICAL DISCLAIMER.

THIS BOOK IS NOT DESIGNED TO, AND DOES NOT, PROVIDE MEDICAL ADVICE. ALL CONTENT ("CONTENT"), INCLUDING TEXT, GRAPHICS, IMAGES AND INFORMATION AVAILABLE ON OR THROUGHOUT THIS BOOK ARE FOR GENERAL INFORMATIONAL PURPOSES ONLY GAINED THROUGH THE AUTHORS EXTENSIVE RESEARCH AND EXPERIENCES.

THE CONTENT IS NOT INTENDED TO BE A SUBSTITUTE FOR PROFESSIONAL MEDICAL ADVICE, DIAGNOSIS OR TREATMENT. NEVER DISREGARD PROFESSIONAL MEDICAL ADVICE, OR DELAY IN SEEKING IT, BECAUSE OF SOMETHING YOU HAVE READ IN THIS BOOK. NEVER RELY ON INFORMATION IN THIS BOOK IN PLACE OF SEEKING PROFESSIONAL MEDICAL ADVICE.

THE AUTHOR IS NOT RESPONSIBLE OR LIABLE FOR ANY ADVICE, COURSE OF TREATMENT, DIAGNOSIS OR ANY OTHER INFORMATION, SERVICES OR PRODUCTS THAT YOU OBTAIN THROUGH THIS BOOK. YOU ARE ENCOURAGED TO CONFER WITH YOUR DOCTOR WITH REGARD TO INFORMATION CONTAINED IN OR THROUGH THIS BOOK. AFTER READING THE CONTENT FROM THIS BOOK, YOU ARE ENCOURAGED TO REVIEW THE INFORMATION CAREFULLY WITH YOUR PROFESSIONAL HEALTHCARE PROVIDER.

July-2014 SN Paleo ©.

printedition 2014 ©.

Made in the USA
Middletown, DE
05 September 2017